Eva Schmidt

**SEXUALITY & PARTNERSHIP IN HUNTINGTON'S DISEASE AND MULTIPLE SCLEROSIS**

Eva Schmidt

# SEXUALITY & PARTNERSHIP IN HUNTINGTON'S DISEASE AND MULTIPLE SCLEROSIS

The impact of Huntington's disease and Multiple Sclerosis on Partnership, Sexual Behavior and Body Image

Südwestdeutscher Verlag für Hochschulschriften

**Impressum/Imprint (nur für Deutschland/ only for Germany)**
Bibliografische Information der Deutschen Nationalbibliothek: Die Deutsche Nationalbibliothek verzeichnet diese Publikation in der Deutschen Nationalbibliografie; detaillierte bibliografische Daten sind im Internet über http://dnb.d-nb.de abrufbar.
Alle in diesem Buch genannten Marken und Produktnamen unterliegen warenzeichen-, markenoder patentrechtlichem Schutz bzw. sind Warenzeichen oder eingetragene Warenzeichen der jeweiligen Inhaber. Die Wiedergabe von Marken, Produktnamen, Gebrauchsnamen, Handelsnamen, Warenbezeichnungen u.s.w. in diesem Werk berechtigt auch ohne besondere Kennzeichnung nicht zu der Annahme, dass solche Namen im Sinne der Warenzeichen- und Markenschutzgesetzgebung als frei zu betrachten wären und daher von jedermann benutzt werden dürften.

Verlag: Südwestdeutscher Verlag für Hochschulschriften Aktiengesellschaft & Co. KG
Dudweiler Landstr. 99, 66123 Saarbrücken, Deutschland
Telefon +49 681 37 20 271-1, Telefax +49 681 37 20 271-0, Email: info@svh-verlag.de
Zugl.: Graz, Medical University, Diss., 2007

Herstellung in Deutschland:
Schaltungsdienst Lange o.H.G., Berlin
Books on Demand GmbH, Norderstedt
Reha GmbH, Saarbrücken
Amazon Distribution GmbH, Leipzig
ISBN: 978-3-8381-0626-7

**Imprint (only for USA, GB)**
Bibliographic information published by the Deutsche Nationalbibliothek: The Deutsche Nationalbibliothek lists this publication in the Deutsche Nationalbibliografie; detailed bibliographic data are available in the Internet at http://dnb.d-nb.de.
Any brand names and product names mentioned in this book are subject to trademark, brand or patent protection and are trademarks or registered trademarks of their respective holders. The use of brand names, product names, common names, trade names, product descriptions etc. even without a particular marking in this works is in no way to be construed to mean that such names may be regarded as unrestricted in respect of trademark and brand protection legislation and could thus be used by anyone.

Publisher:
Südwestdeutscher Verlag für Hochschulschriften Aktiengesellschaft & Co. KG
Dudweiler Landstr. 99, 66123 Saarbrücken, Germany
Phone +49 681 37 20 271-1, Fax +49 681 37 20 271-0, Email: info@svh-verlag.de

Copyright © 2009 by the author and Südwestdeutscher Verlag für Hochschulschriften Aktiengesellschaft & Co. KG and licensors
All rights reserved. Saarbrücken 2009

Printed in the U.S.A.
Printed in the U.K. by (see last page)
ISBN: 978-3-8381-0626-7

# Table of contents

1. INTRODUCTION  5

   1.1. Reasons for choosing the topic of sexuality in HD and MS ..........5

   1.2. Huntington's disease ..........7

   1.3. Multiple sclerosis ..........8

      1.3.1. Diagnostic Criteria ..........9

   1.4. Sexuality in general ..........12

   1.5. Sexual dysfunction ..........13

      1.5.1. Paraphilia. ..........13

      1.5.2. The central nervous system and sexuality ..........13

      1.5.3. Reasons for sexual disorders. ..........14

   1.6. Treatment options for sexual dysfunction in general ..........14

   1.7. Sexual dysfunction in chronic diseases ..........15

      1.7.1. Mechanism of sexual dysfunction ..........15

      1.7.2. Relationship between sexual disorder and level of disability. ..........16

      1.7.3. Stroke and sexual dysfunction. ..........16

   1.8. Sexuality in Huntington's disease ..........17

      1.8.1. Hypersexuality ..........17

      1.8.2. Hyposexuality ..........17

      1.8.3. Studies and limitations ..........18

      1.8.4. Behavioral changes and sexual dysfunction ..........19

      1.8.5. Cerebral dysfunction and sexuality ..........19

      1.8.6. Hormones and sexuality ..........20

      1.8.7. Treatment options ..........20

   1.9. Sexuality in patients with Multiple sclerosis ..........21

      1.9.1. Studies on sexuality and MS ..........21

      1.9.2. Sexual dysfunction in men with MS ..........22

      1.9.3. Sexual dysfunction in women with MS ..........22

      1.9.4. Influence of level of bladder functioning ..........22

      1.9.5. Sexual activity, concerning and satisfaction ..........23

      1.9.6. Hypersexuality in MS ..........23

      1.9.7. Partnership and family ..........24

| | | | |
|---|---|---|---|
| | 1.9.8. | Therapeutic approaches for sexual dysfunction | 24 |

## 2. Hypothesis    28

- **2.1. Main Hypothesis** ... 28
- **2.2. Supplementary hypotheses** ... 28
  - 2.2.1. Differences in sexual dysfunction ... 28
  - 2.2.2. Differences in sexual activities ... 28
  - 2.2.3. Differences in body image and self confidence ... 28
  - 2.2.4. Differences in relationship satisfaction ... 29
- **2.3. Null hypothesis** ... 29

## 3. Patients and Methods    30

- **3.1. Recruiting of patients** ... 30
  - 3.1.1. Course of investigations ... 30
  - 3.1.2. Recruiting of MS patients ... 30
  - 3.1.3. Recruiting of HD patients ... 31
  - 3.1.4. Exclusion criteria ... 31
- **3.2. Questionnaires and Problems** ... 31
  - 3.2.1. Standardized questionnaires ... 34
  - 3.2.2. The personal interview ... 38

## 4. General data and analysis 39

- **4.1. General problems** ... 39
- **4.2. Sociodemografic data** ... 39
- **4.3. The interview questionnaire „SPCD"** ... 40
  - 4.3.2. "SPCD" analysis ... 41
- **4.4. Standardised questionnaires** ... 43
  - 4.4.1. FLP ... 43
  - 4.4.2. TSST ... 47
  - 4.4.3. FBeK 3-scales ... 48
  - 4.4.4. FBeK 4-scales ... 49
  - 4.4.5. ZIP ... 50
  - 4.4.6. Sexual Functions ... 51
  - 4.4.7. PFB ... 53
  - 4.4.8. PL ... 54

- 4.5. Correlations ................................................................................................................ 54
  - 4.5.1. Correlation between TSST, sum of ZIP, FLP, age and duration of illness ............... 54
  - 4.5.2. Correlation between FBeK, ZIP and SPCD ................................................................ 56
- 4.6. **Case reports** ............................................................................................................ 58
  - 4.6.1. HD patients .................................................................................................................. 58
  - 4.6.2. MS patient ................................................................................................................... 58

# 5. Discussion  59

- 5.1. **Testing of hypotheses** ............................................................................................. 59
  - 5.1.1. Main hypothesis. ......................................................................................................... 59
  - 5.1.2. Supplementary hypothesis ......................................................................................... 60
- 5.2. **Interpretation** ......................................................................................................... 63

# 6. Conclusion  65

# 7. References  66

# 1. INTRODUCTION

## 1.1. Reasons for choosing the topic of sexuality in HD and MS

*Introduction.* Huntington's Disease (HD) and Multiple Sclerosis (MS) are both neurological illnesses progressing either continuously or discontinuously. In addition, severe psychological symptoms resulting from the original illness frequently appear. The illnesses are characterized by their relatively early onset and a disease course that can hardly be influenced by medical treatment despite of substantial progress in research, which poses a serious challenge to affected patients (Calabrese, 2006).

Imagine that most of the patients are in their most productive years- just in progress of having a family on their own or making career, when receiving the diagnosis that they suffer from an in all probability continuous proceeding illness with a more or less unpredictable development. When the patient is confronted with the illness, sexuality is reshaped against a foundation of previous sexual experiences and expectations. As the onset of multiple sclerosis mainly occurs in younger persons between the age of 20 and 40, sexual dysfunctions have great impact on their quality of life (Jonsson, 2003). Constructions of sexuality like physical sexual responses, perceptions of appearance and attractiveness to self and others, communication and relationships, self-image and self-esteem, and the sense of affirmation and acknowledgement that the person experienced from others in his everyday life will influence sexual behaviour and relationship after diagnosis (Koch et al., 2002). The individual experiences a severe alteration in lifestyle both physiologically and emotionally. Suddenly not only the patient himself, but every person in the household has to learn to live with this illness. Each person in the family will see the disease in a different way and therefore family response and coping mechanism cannot be seen as a unified process. If one member becomes unable to carry out his or her particular role, the whole family rhythm can be disturbed (Kalb, 1998). Especially problems with changing roles of a couple can have a great impact on their partnership and sexual life. Unfortunately discussion of alterations in sexuality by health care workers has traditionally been viewed as taboo. Specifically, the sexual concerns in chronic debilitating disorders have been neglected (Csesko, 1988). Sexual dysfunction in HD as well as in MS is a very common problem although it is unclear if it is caused by the chronic illness themselves or by the sociopsychiatric burden. As well it is unexplained if the possible social impact dominates and leads to sexual hypoactive disorder or if organic lesions outweigh causing sexual disinhibited behavior.

There are just a few studies in literature about sexuality in HD. These findings conclude that up to 87% men and up to 75% of women experience high levels of sexual problems, most of them having prevalent symptoms of a hypoactive sexual disorder but also increased sexual interest and paraphilia were found in a high incidence. There is no evidence if sexual dysfunction is mainly a specific symptom of HD and maybe associated with the illness or the specific brain lesion itself or if it is chiefly related to the psychosocial factors caused by the steadily worsening of the disease or by depression itself. The reliability of the hitherto literature is very low, as only one study concerning sexual dysfunction in HD was performed after 1993, though diagnosis was only possible if the patient was already presenting physical symptoms. Thus, the problem is that in most of the studies only severely ill patients were examined. Sexual changes preceding neurological and motor symptoms have not been explored. Therefore our intention was to focus as well on asymptomatic subjects as on patients who already present symptoms to explore general sexual changes.

In contrast to the sparse literature concerning sexuality in HD there is high evidence that people with MS experience high levels of sexual dysfunction most of them with hypoactive sexual behaviour. This is often associated with dissatisfaction in relationship, as also the partners seem to show lower sexual and partnership satisfaction. The most common problems in women are lack of sexual interest and decreased libido, often with problems in orgasmic capacity, while men report erectile dysfunction and also lack of sexual interest. The impact of the level of disability and duration of the illness remains unclear. Positive familial support can often help the patient in coping with his illness; nonetheless problems with changing roles and multiple-sclerosis-minimizing can improve the need of contacts to outstanding persons.

## 1.2. Huntington's disease

Huntington's disease (HD) is an autosomal dominant, inherited, neuropsychiatric disease, which manifests with progressive motor, cognitive and behavioral symptoms with an underlying loss of striatal neurons. On average, symptoms begin between the age of 40 years, in most cases with first more or less nearly inconspicuous movement disorders, proceeding to hyperkinesias of the limbs, uncontrolled movements of facial muscles, dysphagia, dysarthrophonia, tremor and decreased control of the whole muscles, besides psychiatric manifestations as e.g. affectability and, in terminal stages, dementia. The course of HD is steadily progressive, in many cases leading to death after 10-30 years after diagnosis (Lange, 2002). HD is caused by a CAG expansion in the gene encoding the huntingtin (htt) protein which is postulated to result in a toxic gain of protein function together with the elimination of some of the functions of wild-type htt. The degeneration of the basal ganglia, especially the caudate and putamen is caused by a single autosomal gene which leads to a multiplication of the base triplet CAG coding for a mutated form of a protein. In dependence of the number of multiplications, HD can manifest with serious and with apparent symptoms in younger years, or mildly and with late onset. Diagnosis of HD is secure if the patient has 38 or more CAG triplets. Progression of disease is measured by the United Huntington Disease Rating Scale (UHDRS) which is a research tool which has been developed to provide a uniform assessment of the clinical features and course of HD and is used to document changes of the medical condition of the patient. The UHDRS has undergone extensive reliability and validity testing and has been used as a major outcome measure in controlled clinical trials. To state the present clinical condition of the patient one can use the motor section of the UHDRS, whereof the patient in the worst case can gain 124 points, a bettering of symptoms would decrease the score.

Brain size is generally reduced and the striatum, especially the caudate nuclei, early gets atrophic. The severity of the pathology correlates with the gene defect and a longer trinucleotide repeat length is associated with a faster rate of deterioration and greater pathological severity in HD. While the movement disorders in HD that correlates with striatal neuronal loss, is widely explored, the morphological substrate for the cognitive and behavioural decline in HD is controversial and remains unclear. It is variously related to diffuse cortical atrophy with neuron loss and dystrophic neurites leading to disruption of striato-frontal or limbic circuitries (Jellinger, 1998).

Since 1993, direct genetic testing is available, which provides predictive diagnosis even in neurologically asymptomatic persons at risk.

In his original description of HD Georg Huntington wrote about "two married men with HD who are constantly making love to some ladies, not seeming to be aware that there is any impropriety in it and they never let out an opportunity to flirt with a girl" (Craufurd et al., 2001; Huntington,

1872). Changed sexual interest and behavior and sexual dysfunctions are common problems in HD but do not only raise a problem for the patient himself. Also spouses and children suffer from the socio-psychiatric consequences (Dewhurst et al, 1970). The majority of patients are in their most fertile period when they are confronted with the diagnosis of their illness. The deterioration of the disease with hypersexuality and violent behavior often tends to hinder and impair the effectiveness of birth control and they often become demented or irresponsible.

## 1.3. Multiple sclerosis

Multiple Sclerosis (MS), an inflammatory and demyelinating disease, is generally considered solely a neurological disease. So far the real cause of the disease remains widely unknown although most hypothesis point to viral or autoimmune pathogenesis. The disease varies in its course, but in most cases clinical symptoms with motor impairments, sensory deficiencies, optic neuritis, bowel and bladder disturbances are predominant.

In 1868 Jean-Martin Charcot first described MS and since 1870 there have been attempts to identify and diagnose cases of MS in the US. Up to the middle of the 20th century the disease was considered rather rare. Only then did neurologists, above all, start to make the diagnosis of MS more often, probably resulting from improved treatment and training possibilities. Since then MS has been recognized as one of the most widely spread neurological diseases. However, even afterwards there were MS patients being misdiagnosed as suffering from hysteria, neurosyphilis etc. Only for a few years the diagnosis is being made in a relatively certain way with the help of imaging techniques (Talley, 2005). The McDonald criteria are at present the diagnostic criteria for multiple sclerosis. They make use of advances in MRI imaging techniques and facilitate the diagnosis of MS in patients who present with signs and symptoms suggestive of the disease. These include monosymptomatic disease, disease with a typical relapsing-remitting course or insidious progression but no clear attacks and remissions (McDonald et al. 2001; Polman et al. 2005).

But even the psychiatric components of the disease were discovered already at the beginning of the 20$^{th}$ century with affective as well as psychotic symptoms being described in relation to MS. Neuropsychiatric symptoms can often be proved among MS patients as only 30% seem to be stable as far as mental health is concerned, which was clearly confirmed by several scientific studies (Boerner and Kapfhammer, 1999; Feinstein and Feinstein, 2001). The reports mainly point to affective disorders such as Major Depression, bipolar disorders, apathy and euphoria but also to anxiety, personality disorders, pathological laughing and crying and psychoses (Minden and Schiffer, 2000; Minden, 2000; Minden et al., 1987; Nelson et al, 2003; Feinstein et al., 1997, Feinstein et al., 1999, Schmidt et al., 2006).

### 1.3.1. Diagnostic Criteria

*1.3.1.1. Expanded Disability Status Scale (EDSS)*

The Kurtzke Expanded Disability Status Scale (EDSS) is a method of quantifying disability in multiple sclerosis (see Table 1). The EDSS quantifies disability in eight Functional Systems (FS) and allows neurologists to assign a Functional System Score (FSS) in each of these. EDSS steps 1.0 to 4.5 refer to people with MS who are fully ambulatory. EDSS steps 5.0 to 9.5 are defined by the impairment to ambulation. The Functional Systems are:

- pyramidal
- cerebellar
- brainstem
- sensory
- bowel and bladder
- visual
- cerebral
- other

## Table1: Expanded Disability Status Scale (EDSS)

| | |
|---|---|
| 0.0 | Normal neurological examination |
| 1.0 | No disability, minimal signs in one FS |
| 1.5 | No disability, minimal signs in more than one FS |
| 2.0 | Minimal disability in one FS |
| 2.5 | Mild disability in one FS or minimal disability in two FS |
| 3.0 | Moderate disability in one FS, or mild disability in three or four FS. Fully ambulatory |
| 3.5 | Fully ambulatory but with moderate disability in one FS and more than minimal disability in several others |
| 4.0 | Fully ambulatory without aid, self-sufficient, up and about some 12 hours a day despite relatively severe disability; able to walk without aid or rest some 500 meters |
| 4.5 | Fully ambulatory without aid, up and about much of the day, able to work a full day, may otherwise have some limitation of full activity or require minimal assistance; characterized by relatively severe disability; able to walk without aid or rest some 300 meters. |
| 5.0 | Ambulatory without aid/ rest for about 200 m; disability severe enough to impair full daily activities (work a day without special provisions) |
| 5.5 | Ambulatory without aid or rest for about 100 m; disability severe enough to preclude full daily activities |
| 6.0 | Intermittent or unilateral constant assistance (cane, crutch, brace) required to walk about 100 meters with or without resting |
| 6.5 | Constant bilateral assistance (canes, crutches, braces) required to walk about 20 meters without resting |
| 7.0 | Unable to walk beyond approximately five meters even with aid, essentially restricted to wheelchair; wheels self in standard wheelchair and transfers alone; up and about in wheelchair some 12 hours a day |
| 7.5 | Unable to take more than a few steps; restricted to wheelchair; may need aid in transfer; wheels self but cannot carry on in standard wheelchair a full day; May require motorized wheelchair |
| 8.0 | Essentially restricted to bed or chair or perambulated in wheelchair, but may be out of bed itself much of the day; retains many self-care functions; generally has effective use of arms |
| 8.5 | Essentially restricted to bed much of day; has some effective use of arms retains some self care functions |
| 9.0 | Confined to bed; can still communicate and eat. |
| 9.5 | Totally helpless bed patient; unable to communicate effectively or eat/swallow |
| 10.0 | Death due to MS |

### 1.3.1.2. Mc Donald criteria

The McDonald criteria- revised in 2005- are diagnostic criteria for multiple sclerosis that make use of advances in MRI (Magnet Resonance Imaging) techniques (see Table 2). The criteria facilitate the diagnosis of MS in patients who present with signs and symptoms suggestive of the disease.

### Table 2: Mc Donald criteria

| Clinical Presentation | Additional Data Needed |
|---|---|
| • 2 or more attacks (relapses)<br>• 2 or more objective clinical lesions | None; clinical evidence will suffice (additional evidence desirable but must be consistent with MS) |
| • 2 or more attack<br>• 1 objective clinical lesion | Dissemination in space, demonstrated by:<br>➢ MRI<br>➢ or a positive CSF (cerebrospinal fluid) and 2 or more MRI lesions consistent with MS<br>➢ or further clinical attack involving different site |
| • 1 attack<br>• 2 or more objective clinical lesions | Dissemination in time, demonstrated by:<br>➢ MRI<br>➢ or second clinical attack |
| • 1 attack<br>• 1 objective clinical lesion (monosymptomatic presentation) | Dissemination in space by demonstrated by:<br>➢ MRI<br>➢ or positive CSF and 2 or more MRI lesions consistent with MS<br>and dissemination in time demonstrated by:<br>➢ MRI<br>➢ or second clinical attack |
| **Insidious neurological progression suggestive of MS (primary progressive MS)** | One year of disease progression and two of the following:<br>➢ MRI evidence (9 or more T2 brain lesions or four or more T2 lesions with positive VEP)<br>➢ Positive spinal cord MRI (two focal T2 lesions)<br>➢ Positive CSF |

## 1.4. Sexuality in general

Sexuality itself is part of self-identity at any age and can be seen from different points of views. In recent times the priority was given to the reproductive part of sexuality and also in the scientific literature most of the studies focus on clear somatic dysfunction, frequently not noticing the impact of psychosocial factors. Of course, the sexual drive is as old as humanity and evolution itself and necessary for the propagation of all species. However, sexuality is not only influenced by the integrity of the genital tract, also the limbic system and spinal arousal centres are involved (Barton and Joubert, 2000), so sexuality is more than sexual function. It is an ever-changing lived experience and is always affected by the manner in which we view ourselves and our bodies (Hordern et al., 2000), associated with constantly changing social and cultural influences (Barton and Joubert, 2000; Hordern et al., 2000; Bancroft, 1993).

Just lately, with more effective contraception methods and the increasing life expectancy of the whole population, the non-fertile life chapter is getting more and more important. Therefore socio-communicative or relationship-orientated and lust-aspects have an increasing influence on sexual behaviour and the quality of relationship. Sexual satisfaction is more often associated with acceptance, warmth, confidence, open communication, personal security with affiliation to the partner and erotic attraction and passion (Gunzelmann et al., 2004; Weissbach-Rieger, 1987; Loewit, 2003). Therefore, sexual dysfunction- especially among chronically ill people, should not be defined and treated as a clear somatic disorder but under the aspect of cognitive and emotional factors (Chandler and Brown, 1998), helping the patients and their partners to find a new way of their own sexual meanings and partnership (Gunzelmann et al., 2004).

In clinical practice, many physicians feel uncomfortable or inadequately trained to discuss sexual issues with their patients, but the vast majority of patients believe that it is appropriate for physicians to address sexual function within the context of routine health assessment (Vermillion and Holmes, 1997). Also patients very often feel shame and unease when talking directly and frankly about their sexual problems. During the conversation it is most important to find adequate answers to those questions that are merely hidden messages, i.e. to find the right balance between distance and intimacy (Neises, 2002). Asking for sexual concerns and problems will provide the physician with an opportunity to educate patients and furthermore it will give patients the "permission" to address sexual issues in a confidential and non-judgmental setting (see Table 4; Vermillion and Holmes, 1997).

## 1.5. Sexual dysfunction

The term "sexual dysfunction" describes a number of sexual problems that inhibit normal sexual relations and is defined as "disturbances in sexual desire and in the psychophysiological changes that characterize the sexual response cycle and cause marked distress and interpersonal difficulty" (American Psychiatric Association, 1994). However, it should be noted that the lack of standard criteria is an important factor causing problems in the comparison of studies about sexual functioning and dysfunction and that there are inconsistent methods of obtaining information about changes in sexual behavior (see Table 4). There are some studies about the sexual life and the frequency of sexual dysfunctions among the so-called "normal" population. In community samples a current prevalence of up to 10% for female orgasmic disorder, up to 5% for erectile disorder and premature ejaculation and up to 3% for male orgasmic and hypoactive sexual desire disorder has been found (Simons and Carey, 2001). The prevalence of sexual dysfunction in the USA ranges about 31- 43% (Laumann, 1999).

### 1.5.1. Paraphilia.
Paraphilia, also referred as sexual deviation, is described as "persistent or repetitive sexually arousing fantasies of an unusual nature associated with either preference for or use of a nonhuman object for sexual arousal, repetitive sexual activity with human beings involving real or simulated suffering or humiliation, or repetitive sexual activity with non-consenting partners". The diagnosis of a paraphilic disorder is made if a person has acted on the urges or is markedly distressed by them and is an occasional feature of brain diseases (Rich and Ovsiew, 1994).

### 1.5.2. The central nervous system and sexuality.
Sexual responses are under the control of numerous central and peripheral neural systems. The central supraspinal systems are mainly localized in the limbic system, in the hypothalamus and its nuclei. Neural information travels through the brain stem, the medulla oblongata, the spinal cord and the autonomous nervous system to the genital apparatus. Several neurotransmitters and neuropeptides, such as dopamine, glutamic acid, nitric oxide, oxytocin, ACTH-MSH peptides, are known as to facilitate sexual function, while serotonin, gamma-aminobutyric acid (GABA) and opioid peptides reduce it (Argiolas and Melis, 2003). Primary stress hormones especially CRH (corticotropine releasing hormone) also influence sexual activity. Mild stress can sometimes increase sexual urges, sustained stress diminishes sexual urges by producing CRH in the brain which dramatically reduces all prosocial and sexual activities (Panksepp, 2004).

### 1.5.3. Reasons for sexual disorders.

There are different factors influencing sexual functioning and causing sexual disorder. The most important factors are listed as followed. (1) Sexual dysfunction as a consequence of depression. About 50-90% of depressive patients are found to have sexual dysfunctions, comorbidity between sexual dysfunction and depressive illness is high but the causal relationship is unclear (Kasper, 2002). Apart from antidepressant treatment, depression itself may cause a progressive decline in interest in sexual behavior leading to low libido, difficulty in sexual arousal, orgasm problems and frank sexual aversion. The psychosocial distress that often accompanies sexual dysfunction might increase the development of depressive illness, or as some data suggest, depression may cause sexual dysfunction (Seidman, 2002). (2) Sexual dysfunction as a side effect of medical treatment, especially antidepressive treatment with SSRI's, antihypertensives and H2 blockers, can cause sexual dysfunction with decreased libido and erectile dysfunction, but also result in a worsening of pre-existing sexual problems (Fava and Rankin, 2002). (3) Sexual dysfunction can furthermore be caused by a metabolic, cardiovascular, urologic, andrologic and psychiatric illness (Rosen et al., 2003). (4) In addition, cultural, ethnical, social and religious factors can have an impact as well. That is to say, the whole problem in the area of sexual normality and abnormalities is very complex and is related to psychosocial interactions and must be treated individually.

## 1.6. Treatment options for sexual dysfunction in general

Guidelines for sexual problems in the normal population refer to sildenafil, vardenafil and tadalafil, as first line therapy for male sexual dysfunction especially for erectile disorders (DasGupta and Fowler, 2003). Although awareness of female sexual dysfunction is increasing, there are still just some therapy trials available like estrogen replacement therapy or also sildenafil to support muscle relaxation (Laan et al., 2001; Kaplan et al., 1999). In a recent review medications for the treatment of hypersexuality and paraphilic disorder are categorized into two main groups: the testosterone-lowering agents (i.e., progesterone derivatives and the gonadotropin-releasing hormones (GNRHs) and the serotonergic antidepressants (serotonin-specific reuptake inhibitors) (Saleh and Guidry, 2003). Medroxyprogesterone acetate- (MPA), leuprolide, a gonadotropine-releasing hormone (GnRH) agonist and Cyproterone acetate (CPA) maybe useful to decrease sexually deviant fantasies and urges and eliminate sex-offending behavior by decreasing plasma levels of testosterone and influencing hypothalamic neurons (Gagne, 1981; Rich and Ovsiew, 1994; Krueger and Kaplan, 2001). SSRI's have have been studied in these disorders in an uncontrolled way but appear promising (Krueger and Kaplan, 2001). Psychosocial and cognitve-behavioral approaches should address the intricate biopsychosocial influences of the patient, the partner, and the couple.

Assessment sexual dysfunction should ideally include inquiry about: predisposing, precipitating, maintaining, and contextual factors but in many cases, neither psychotherapy alone nor medical intervention alone is sufficient for the lasting resolution of sexual problems.

Psychotherapeutic strategies in the treatment of sex offenders appear to have positive effects in reducing sex-offending recidivism (Saleh and Guidry, 2003). However e.g. patients with HD are limited in their capacity to sustain behavioral changes relative to their variable mental statuses. As with all- especially pharmacological- treatments, the choice of which drug to use should be based on the presenting symptoms, the concomitant psychiatric conditions, and a thorough review of the patient's psychosexual and medical history.

## 1.7. Sexual dysfunction in chronic diseases

The connection between sexual dysfunction and illness is a very complicated, one, which usually results from a complex interaction of biological, psychological and social factors and can therefore be strongly influenced by one's own sense of self and social competence (Barton and Joubert, 2000). Sexual dysfunction is often reported in chronic diseases. Although not life-threatening, it is associated with a considerable amount of unhappiness and decreasedquality of life (7.0% to 24.2% lower than among people without sexual dysfunction) {Weissbach-Rieger, 1987; Chandler and Brown, 1998; Janardhan and Bakshi, 2002; McKee and Schover, 2001; Perez et al., 2002; Rice, 2000; Ventegodt, 1996; Zlotta and Schulmann, 1999).

### 1.7.1. Mechanism of sexual dysfunction.

The mechanism of interference may be of neurological, vascular, endocrinological, musculoskeletal, or psychological nature and is influenced by many different factors, such as psychosocial environment, including family and religious background, the sexual partner, and individual factors such as self-concept and self-esteem (Nusbaum et al., 2003). Furthermore, people with sexual dysfunctions usually suffer from a combination of organic and psychogenic problems and there are also certain causes for psychic problems such as partnership or personality (Kockott, 1989). Another interesting aspect associated with illness, partnership and sexuality is that younger people e.g. suffering from breast cancer are more often affected by severe emotional distress than older patients although younger ones can expect a better prognosis regarding medical treatment (Schover, 1994). Consistent with findings from studies with general community samples, older people reported significantly fewer depressive symptoms than younger patients with MS (Kneebone et al., 2003). Announcing the findings of a study with 14.009 MS-patients, the majority of depressed and more affected patients was female and younger than other MS patients. In addition most of them had unsettled relationships and tended to be slightly less disabled (Buchanan et al., 2003). Maybe the reason for it is that nowadays, appearance and physical attractiveness play a more important role, especially among young people and therefore, young MS patients often feel more irritated by the possibly disabling and unpredictable development of their illness, which can slightly influence their partnership and whole lifestyle.

### 1.7.2. Relationship between sexual disorder and level of disability.

Focussing on the impact of chronic illnesses on sexuality the study of McCabe and Taleporos investigated in 2003 the association between the severity and duration of physical disability and sexual esteem, sexual depression, sexual satisfaction, and the frequency of sexual behaviour. 1,196 participants completed the study of whom 748 participants (367 males and 381 females) had a physical disability and 448 participants (171 males and 277 females) were able-bodied (their age ranging between 18-69 years, with an average age of 36.39 years). The results demonstrate that people with more severe physical impairments experienced significantly lower levels of sexual esteem and sexual satisfaction and significantly higher levels of sexual depression and were sexual active less frequently. Women with physical disabilities had significantly more positive feelings about their sexuality and significantly more frequent mutual sexual experiences than the male counterparts. People who had experienced their physical impairment for a longer period of time reported significantly more positive feelings about their sexuality (McCabe and Taleporos, 2003).

### 1.7.3. Stroke and sexual dysfunction.

Similarly, studies on patients after stroke showed a high increase in sexual dysfunction and erectile and orgasmic dysfunction was frequent. Decreases in different kinds of affectionate behaviour and dissatisfaction were frequent and half of the patients felt a worsening of the sexual partnership responsiveness. The high prevalence of sexual dysfunction in stroke victims was not associated with endocrine or treatment issues and appeared mostly to be psychogenic. A lack of sexual information and counselling may contribute to the deterioration of partnership sexuality (Sjogren I, 1983; Sjogren II, 1983) and may in a high rate be a reason for changes in role function and increased dependency on the partner (Burgener and Logan, 1989).

## 1.8. Sexuality in Huntington's disease

Only few studies have tried to explore sexuality and sexual dysfunction in HD. Dating back to 1966 until July 2006 on studies dealing with "sexuality", "Huntington", "Huntington's disease", "chorea", "sexual", and "fertility" in the Medline just five studies can be found including a minimum sample of 20 patients allowing for statistical conclusions and providing complete description of the study population (see Table 3) (Bolt, 1970, Craufurd et al., 2001; Dewhurst et al., 1970; Fedoroff et al., 1994; Oliver, 1970). The major finding of the few studies that have tried to explore sexuality and sexual dysfunction in HD is a high frequency of sexual disorders in patients with HD (Schmidt et al., 2007). The most frequent sexual disorder reported was hypoactive sexual behavior although increased sexual interest and paraphilia were found in a high incidence. All of the studies reported on sexual dysfunction in patients with HD. The prevalence was ranging up to 85% in men and 75% in women (Fedoroff et al., 1994).

### 1.8.1. Hypersexuality

Hypersexual behavior was more prevalent in men ranging from 3.9 % to 30 %, in women from 2.1 % to 25 %. Dewhurst et al. reported in his study of the socio-psychiatric consequences of HD that 30 of 102 patients displayed abnormal sexual behavior, of whom 19 (18.6%) showed hypersexuality (Dewhurst et al., 1970). Bolt found that only 20 (6%) of 334 patients had increased libido or sexual deviation and Oliver also reported 6% of the patients displaying similar behaviors (Bolt, 1970; Oliver, 1970). Recent studies reported that 30 % of the HD males and 25 % of the HD females had experienced increased sexual interest (Fedoroff et al., 1994). 134 patients attending an HD management clinic were interviewed by Craufurd et al. in 2001 (Craufurd et al., 2001), using the Problem Behavior Assessment for HD (PBA-HD). Uninhibited sexual behavior was reported by 6 % of the patients by Craufurd et al. while demanding or persistent sexual behavior was described in 5 %. Interestingly, only this study sought to determine changes in sexual interest with behavioral changes. Hypersexual behavior was associated with a behavioral profile characterized by irritability, mental inflexibility and obsessive-compulsive or perseverative behaviors (Craufurd et al., 2001).

### 1.8.2. Hyposexuality

In opposite to those findings some studies reported that loss of libido and hyposexuality are much more common in HD. Decreased sexual interest was found between 6.9% and 63% in men and in 3.9% to 75 % in women. In two studies there were no data concerning hyposexuality applicable (Bolt, 1970; Oliver, 1970). Fedoroff et al. reported that 63% of a sample of 27 HD males and 75%

of the 12 females showed a hypoactive sexual disorder, 56% and 42% had inhibited orgasm. The most remarkable finding of Fedoroff et al. was the very high frequency of inhibited male orgasm. In this study significantly more men who had as well problems withinhibited orgasm as an increased sexual interest also had paraphilic disorders (Fedoroff et al., 1994). 134 patients attending an HD management clinic were interviewed by Craufurd et al. in 2001, using the Problem Behavior Assessment for HD (Craufurd et al., 2001). Loss of libido was reported in 61.8 % of patients and correlated significantly with the PBA-HD score and inversely with Total Function Capacity score. Another interesting aspect is that patient's wives often complained that their husbands were demanding an inordinate amount of sexual fulfillment at odd times or at inadequate places and whenever these desires were refused they became violent and abusive (Dewhurst et al., 1970). Sexual problems in the partners of HD patients were also reported in a more recent study. 32 partners were interviewed by Fedoroff et al. and showed in 66% one or more sexualdisorders by DSM-III-R criteria (Fedoroff et al., 1994) but there was a numerically greater frequency of paraphilia in the HD cases than in their partners (19 % of HD males versus 10 % of the non HD males; 8 % of the HD females versus 0 % of the non HD females) (Fedoroff et al., 1994).

### 1.8.3. Studies and limitations

Different authors used different strategies in recruiting HD patients, most of them provided retrospective explorations or described the life time prevalence of sexual problems in HD (Bolt, 1970; Oliver, 1970; Dewhurst et al., 1970; Tyler) only two conducted direct interview in clinic waiting rooms (Fedoroff et al., 1994; Craufurd et al., 2001). Evidence of sexual dysfunction was either based on personal information of the patient himself, on statements of partners and family members or on diagnosis by medical doctors and therefore renders the results difficult to compare. As only one study concerning sexual dysfunction in HD was performed after 1993, diagnosis was only possible if the patient was already presenting physical symptoms. Thus, the problem is that in most of the studies only severely ill patients were examined. Only one study interviewed both the patients and their partners and explored the agreement between them (Fedoroff et al., 1994). Couples were found to be more likely to agree on the absence of a particular disorder than on its presence and leads to the assumption that participants more likely underreport than overreport sexual problems. Moreover, psychosocial factors influencing sexual behavior such as stability of partnership and marriage or breakup of relationships are not further explored in the present surveys, just Dewhurst et al. in 1970 reports a break up of 38% of marriages (Dewhurst et al., 1970).
An interesting finding of Fedoroff et al. is that men who have as well problems with inhibited orgasm as an increased sexual interest more often show paraphilic disorders (Fedoroff et al., 1994). Possibly sexual problems in patients and their partners are partially caused and aggravated by the

mismatch of present sexual desire but the impossibility of acting out these feelings. The age of the population was ranging between twenty and more than eighty years; in some studies the exact range of the age of the patients interviewed on sexuality was not even described. Most of them did retrospective explorations or describe the life time prevalence of sexual problems in HD (Bolt, 1970; Oliver, 1970; Dewhurst et al., 1970; Tyler) only two provided direct interviews in clinic waiting rooms (Fedoroff et al., 1994; Craufurd et al., 2001). Only Fedoroff et al. interviewed both the patients and their partners and explored the agreement between them (Fedoroff et al., 1994). This study is also the only one just focusing on sexual dysfunction in HD, all the others were exploring neuropsychiatric or behavioral changes, finding sexual dysfunction as a prominent symptom.

### 1.8.4. Behavioral changes and sexual dysfunction

Only one study tried to associate behavioral changes with sexual dysfunction (Craufurd et al., 2001). Hypersexual behavior was associated with a behavioral profile characterized by irritability, mental inflexibility and obsessive-compulsive or perseverative behaviors. Suggestions for possible mechanism causing sexual dysfunction were barely discussed but we know that damage to cortical areas may worsen sexual functioning by influencing concentration and thinking (Fedoroff et al., 1994). Damage to cortical areas may worsen sexual functioning by influencing concentration and thinking (Fedoroff et al., 1994).

### 1.8.5. Cerebral dysfunction and sexuality

Damage to the striatum may play a role in inhibited orgasm by interrupting motor patterns but similarly by changing dopaminergic and serotonergic pathways in patients with HD which have been implicated in the regulation of sex hormones (Markianos et al, 2005; Fedoroff et al., 1994). The striatum receives both dopaminergic and serotonergic input and many striatal local circuit neurons are cholinergic. In addition different biochemical processes and a n atrophy of the dienzephalon may be involved. Mice models of HD suggest that the characteristic striatal neuropathology and testicular degeneration in HD is caused primarily by the toxicity of mutant huntingtin (Van Raamsdonk et al, 2005). This large protein of uncertain function is ubiquitously expressed in many tissues of the body but is at highest levels in brain and testis (Leavitt et al, 2001). In animal models an inactivation of the Huntington disease gene resulted in male sterility due to reduced sperm production (Dragastsis et al, 2000). In addition atrophy of the reproductive organs, reduced testicular mass and loss of fertility have been observed in mice models of HD (Papalexi et al, 2005). As a normal breeding behavior could be noticed, a defect in spermatogenesis is suggested to be responsible for the lack of fertility (Leavitt et al, 2001). Further, it is assumed that the spermatogenetic defect is not caused by a defective maturation or limited to a single stage of development of spermatocytes, as degenerating cells at various stages of development were identified in animal models (Leavitt et al, 2001; Papalexi et al, 2005).

### 1.8.6. Hormones and sexuality

A reduction of circulating testosterone level in male HD patients (Markianos et al, 2005) and decreased expression of gonatropine-releasing hormone (GnRH) in the hypothalamus and blood testosterone level (Papalexi et al, 2005) together with atrophy of gonads and sterility in transgenic mice model of HD (Sathasivam et al, 1999; Dragatsis et al, 2000; Leavitt et al, 2001; Papalexi et al, 2005; Van Raamsdonk et al, 2005) is described.

Not only in male mice models but also in male HD patients testosterone levels were significantly lower compared to healthy men suggesting the influence of GnRH, athough this increase is not accompanied by a reduction in luteinizing hormone (LH) levels (Markianos et al, 2005). Thus, the reduction in testosterone might be caused by the reduced dopaminergic input to pituitary, possibly because of a loss of hypothalamic dopaminergic and GnRH neurons (Markianos et al, 2005; Papalexi et al, 2005). Also the physiological basis of sexual behavior in female HD patients indicates changes in concentration of GnRH (Bird et al, 1976). Infertility could be due to death of GnRH neurons or to a reduction in GnRH expression leading to a downstream impairment of the gonadotropic hormones (Papalexi et al, 2005). The direct neural hypothalamic- testicular pathway interferes with synthesis and secretion of testosterone in the Leydig cells independent of pituitary. This could explain the great reductions in testosterone in patients with severe symptomatology, in whom LH levels were found to be normal (Markianos et al, 2005). Interestingly, although reduced testosterone levels are known to cause loss in muscle mass, testosterone treatment had no effect on body weight loss and did not restore motor function in transgenic HD mice (Papalexi et al, 2005).

Estrogens and derivates have been shown to protect neurons from oxidative stress-induced death in animal models and could have a beneficial effect in HD but did not induce modification in motor disabilities (Tunez et al, 2006; Bonuc(c)elli et al, 1992).

### 1.8.7. Treatment options

Treatment options for HD patients with sexual disorder have yet not been studied in detail and are only reported sporadically, guidelines can only be obtained from non-HD patients and further research is needed.

## 1.9. Sexuality in patients with Multiple sclerosis

Sexual dysfunction in MS is described as having three basic influence factors. First of all, sexual dysfunctions occur as a result of multiple-sclerosis -related, neurological changes that directly affect sexual feelings and/or sexual response. The most common symptoms are decreased libido, altered genital sensation, decreased vaginal lubrication and decreased frequency or intensity of orgasm. Secondary sexual dysfunctions are multiple sclerosis-related physical changes, which affect the sexual response indirectly and are caused by multiple sclerosis symptoms that do not directly include nervous system pathways related to the genital system. Fatigue, muscle tightness, weakness, spasms, bladder and bowel dysfunction, bad coordination, difficulties with mobility, side effects of multiple sclerosis medication, cognitive difficulties, numbness, pain, burning, or discomfort in non-genital areas of the body seem to be most common. The so-called tertiary sexual dysfunction is caused by psychological, emotional, social, and cultural aspects of multiple sclerosis that impact sexuality such as negative changes in self-image, mood, or body-image, depression and anger, feeling less sexy or attractive, fear of being rejected sexually, difficulties in communicating with one's partner, fear of isolation and abandonment, guilt, changing gender roles, and feelings of dependency (See Table 4) (Jonsson, 2003; Foley and Sanders, 1997).

Depression in literature- as one important symptom of tertiary sexual dysfunction is found to be in a very high rate associated with multiple sclerosis (Fruehwald et al., 2001; Zephir et al., 2003; Avasarala et al, 2003; Patten et al., 2003; Solari et al., 2004). Significant correlations with depression and sexual dysfunction have also been found in other chronic illness (e.g. among Diabetes patients), supporting a causative role of psychological factors for sexual problems (Janardhan and Bakshi, 2002; Buvat and Lemmaire, 2001; Monga et al., 1998). Apart from antidepressive treatment, depression itself may cause a progressive decline in interest in sexual behaviour leading to low libido, difficulty in sexual arousal, orgasm problems and frank sexual aversion (Graziottin, 1998), while anxiety was found to have the most important influence on reduced frequency of intercourse (Channon and Ballinger, 1986). Fatigue is one of the most commonly occurring secondary sexual symptoms among people with the illness (e. g. among Diabetes patients), and can significantly interfere with sexual desire and the physical ability to initiate and sustain sexual activity (Valleroy et al., 1984).

### 1.9.1. Studies on sexuality and MS

In the hitherto literature there are and have been many studies on different health related subjects connected with Multiple sclerosis but very few facing sexuality and multiple sclerosis (see Table 5). The ones to be found in literature are in most cases related to clear somatic sexual dysfunction e.g.

descriptions of the pathophysiology of erectile dysfunction or the pharmacological management of erectile dysfunction in men, and not so much to partnership influences or family interactions (Schmidt et al., 2005).

### 1.9.2. Sexual dysfunction in men with MS

Sexual changes and dysfunctions among men were in all studies found among multiple sclerosis patients. The highest result, reported by Lilius et al (Lilius et al., 1976), was about 91%, followed by 78% (Mattson et al., 1995), 75% by Valleroy and Kraft (Valleroy et al., 1984), same as by Jonsson (Jonsson, 2003) and 64% by McCabe (McCabe et al., 1996). Most common are erectile dysfunction, ranging from19 to 62% (Jonsson, 2003; Valleroy et al., 1984; Mattson et al., 1995; Lilius et al., 1976; McCabe et al., 1996), reduced libido, problems achieving orgasm (including premature and retarded ejaculation) and decreased sensation. Also reduced frequency of masturbation is reported (McCabe et al., 1996). In recent studies a significant difference in sexual functioning between the male general population and male multiple sclerosis patients was proved while females with multiple sclerosis only differed from females from the general population in their levels of masturbation and numbness of the genital area (McCabe, 2002).

### 1.9.3. Sexual dysfunction in women with MS

Other experts report sexual female dysfunction among multiple sclerosis patients as being a bit lower than in men, ranging from nearly 80% (McCabe et al., 1996), to 72% by Lilius (Lilius et al., 1976) and to less frequent occurrence with about more or less 50% (Jonsson, 2003; Valleroy et al., 1984; Mattson et al., 1995). Loss of, or problems achieving orgasm and reduced libido are common reported difficulties and appeared among 24 to nearly 60% of the patients (Jonsson, 2003; Valleroy et al., 1984; Mattson et al., 1995; Lilius et al., 1976; McCabe et al., 1996; Hulter et al., 1995). Also sensory genital dysfunction- in 61% - and decreased vaginal lubrication- ranging from 20 to 36%; are frequent sexual dysfunctions among female MS patients (Jonsson, 2003; Mattson et al., 1995; McCabe et al., 1996; Hulter et al., 1995).

### 1.9.4. Influence of level of bladder functioning

On the whole, the sexually less active or inactive patients were different from the as-active-as-before-MS patients in various ways, but most significantly were their difficulties with toilet transfer and bladder functioning (Szasz et al., 1984), which is also confirmed by Valleroy& Kraft and Hulter& Lundberg, who also, according to many other studies in literature, showed an association between bladder functioning and sexual function (Valleroy and Kraft, 1984; Hulter and Lundberg, 1995; Fowler, 1997).

### 1.9.5. Sexual activity, concerning and satisfaction

Szasz et al. found that among 73 men and women with MS, 45% of the researched patients were sexually less active since they developed MS and that only 27% of the group were concerned about the change (Szasz et al., 1984). This is also shown by the study of McCabe where the majority- 53,5%- of respondents with multiple sclerosis, were not concerned or were only a bit concerned about their sexual difficulties (McCabe et al., 1996). Perhaps people with multiple sclerosis accept sexual dysfunction as a symptom of their disorder and feel there is nothing that they can do about this problem, and so do not become overly concerned. Alternatively, some people with MS may now regard kissing, embracing, caressing, and to a lesser extent manual and oral-genital contact as appropriate substitutes for intercourse. Patients in different studies also reported a substantial change to the range and frequency of sexual activities since the development of multiple sclerosis. The incidence of sexual intercourse was low and in most cases less than before multiple sclerosis and was reported by 45%, to two thirds of the respondents of one study group (experiencing intercourse just once a month or less) and up till 80% in the study of Lilius in 1976 (Szasz et al., 1984; McCabe et al., 1996; Lilius et al., 1976). The patients themselves but also their healthy partners experienced low levels of satisfaction with their sexual functions and described that communication, caresses and expressing feelings correlated with better sexual satisfaction (McCabe et al., 2003; McCabe et al., 1996; Beier et al., 2002). In contrast to these findings, McCabe explained in 2002 that although coping strategies and levels of cognitive functioning are important predictors of sexual satisfaction, sexual dysfunction, and relationship satisfaction especially for women with MS, but there were fewer coping or health-related factors that predicted these variables among men with multiple sclerosis (McCabe, 2002). Other results also suggest that strategies, used to cope with the illness, may not play a role in sexual and relationship satisfaction (McCabe et al., 2003). In contrast to the findings of Valleroy and Kraft (Valleroy and Kraft, 1984), Stenager et al. (Stenager et al., 1990), Mattson (Mattson et al., 1995) and McCabe (McCabe et al., 1996), Beier et al. (Beier et al., 2002), that there is no correlation between the level of disability and sexual dysfunction, Szasz et al. (Szasz et al., 1984) and Hulter & Lundberg (Hulter and Lundberg, 1995) found that patients with higher levels of disability experienced greater problems with their sexual functioning. The impact of level of disability on sexual dysfunction therefore remains unclear.

### 1.9.6. Hypersexuality in MS

Although most studies have been focused on a decrease in sexual functioning as a result of MS, this may not always be the case (McCabe et al., 1996). Huws et al. reported that hypersexuality and fetishism appeared in a patient with multiple sclerosis suggesting that the organic neuropsychological effects of multiple sclerosis may extend to sexual behaviour (Huws et al., 1991). Surprisingly, it is also reported that corticosteroid treatment, started for problems other than sexual dysfunction, resulted in improved sexual functioning in many patients (Mattson et al., 1995) while other authors found it to have a negative impact on the sexual functioning of the patients (Beier et al., 2002).

### 1.9.7. Partnership and family

Sexual function frequently relies for its expression on the presence and cooperation of a partner (McCabe et al., 1996). We know that multiple sclerosis results in increasing dependence upon others for both social and practical support. Because the family is often the closest and obvious source of this support, the development of multiple sclerosis has a significant effect on family dynamics. The increased dependence, especially on the partner- often with changing roles, can be a big strain on relationships although high levels of social support may assist in the adjustment of people with multiple sclerosis to the illness (De Loach et al., 1981). McCabe reported, that since developing multiple sclerosis, about one third of respondents had a relationship breakdown or more distant relationship, about one third indicated that their relationships were closer, and about one third indicated no change in their relationships- so relationships seem to remain strong (McCabe et al., 1996), although many of the sexual dysfunctioning patients reported associated marital problems (Mattson et al., 1995). In addition, patients often have better interactions with friends than with the close family members (Dakof et a., 1990) because the recipients may not always view the too close social support as being appropriate. Expressions of concern, love, and understanding were regarded as the most helpful behaviours, whereas minimizing or maximizing the effect of multiple sclerosis and its associated symptoms were seen as the most un-helpful responses. The problem of minimization is particularly relevant for people with multiple sclerosis, because they mostly still "look well" although they may be experiencing substantial symptoms from the illness (Lehman et al., 1990).

### 1.9.8. Therapeutic approaches for sexual dysfunction

Therapeutic principles have shown that first line therapy for male sexual dysfunction especially for erectile disorders is sildenafil, which leads to smooth muscle relaxation and thus erection by releasing NO. Newer phoshpodiesterase 5 inhibitors like vardenafil and tadalafil are similar in the mechanism of action but with different speed of onset and longer duration of effect (DasGupta et al., 2003). Although awareness of female sexual dysfunction is increasing, there are still just some therapy trials available like estrogen replacement therapy to improve vaginal dryness, burning and dyspareunia or also sildenafil to support muscle relaxation (Laan et al., 2001; Kaplan et al., 1999).

## Table 3: Sexuality in Huntington's disease

| Author | Number of patients | Sexual dysfunction | Prevalent paraphilia |
|---|---|---|---|
| Dewhurst (1970) | 102 | 29,4% <br> Hyper-sexual: 18,6% (19) <br> 11,8% ♂; 6,9% ♀ <br> Hypo-sexual: 10,8% (11) <br> 6,9% ♂; 3,9% ♀ | Morbid sexual jealousy, indecent exposure, homosexual assault, incestuous sodomy, voyeurism, assault on females, promiscuity |
| Oliver (1970) | 100 | Hyper-sexual: 6% <br> Hypo-sexual: n.a. | uncontrolled sexual advances sodomy, incest, masturbation in front of own children |
| Bolt (1970) | 334 | Hyper-sexual: 6% <br> 3,9% ♂; 2,1% ♀ <br> Hypo-sexual: n.a. | Increased libido, indicent exposure, children perversity |
| Tyler | 92 | 23% ♂; 9% ♀ <br> Hyper-sexual: 6,5% <br> Hypo-sexual: 7,6% | n.a. |
| Fedoroff (1994) | 39 | 85% ♂; 75% ♀ <br> Hyper-sexual: <br> 30% ♂; 25% ♀ <br> Hypo-sexual: <br> 63% ♂; 75% ♀ | Transsexualism, exhibitionism, increase in sexual interest, obscene phone calls, incestuous thoughts |
| Craufurd (2001) | 134 | Hyper-sexual: <br> 6% sexual disinhibition <br> 5% sexually demanding behavior <br> Hypo-sexual: 62% | n.a. |

n.a.: not applicable

**Table 4: Details taking the sexual history of MS patients**

| **Questions to explore sexual function** |
|---|
| (Nicolosi et al., 2004; Rosen et al., 1997) |
| • Changes in sexual interests and desire |
| • Changes in sexual arousal |
| • Ability to achieve orgasm |
| • Changes in sexual satisfaction |
| • for men: early ejaculation and erection difficulties |

| **Other factors influencing sexual functioning** |
|---|
| (Clayton, 2001; Kalayjian et al., 2000) |
| • Other medical illness (hypertension, diabetes, thyroid diseases, endocrine disorders, neurological disease…) |
| • psychiatric illnesses |
| • evaluation of medications and/or other substances taken (antihypertensives, H2 blockers, antidepressants..) |
| • bladder/ bowel disturbances |
| • personal cultural, religious, social and ethnic background |

**Table 5: Sexuality in Multiple Sclerosis**

| Author | Sexual dysfunction | Dominant sexual dysfunction women | Dominant sexual dysfunction men |
|---|---|---|---|
| **Lilius 1976** | ➢ Women 72%<br>➢ Men 91% | • loss of orgasm (33%)<br>• loss of libido (27%)<br>• spastic (12%) | • erectile dysfunction (62%) |
| **Valleroy & Kraft 1984** | ➢ Women 56%<br>➢ Men 75% | • fatigue<br>• decreased sensation<br>• decreased libido<br>• orgasm problems | • erectile dysfunction<br>• decreased sensation<br>• fatigue<br>• decreased libido<br>• orgasmic dysfunction |
| **Mattson 1995** | ➢ Women 45%<br>➢ Men 78% | • Poor vaginal lubrication<br>• decreased sensation<br>• orgasm problems | • erectile dysfunction<br>• decreased sensation<br>• orgasm problems |
| **Hulter & Lundberg 1995** | | • sensory genital dysfunction (61%)<br>• lack of sexual interest (59%)<br>• orgasmic problems (38%)<br>• poor lubri-cation (36%) | |
| **McCabe 1996** | ➢ Women 79%<br>➢ Men 64% | • lack of sexual interest (29%)<br>• orgasm problems (23.7%)<br>• poor lubrication (19.4%) | • erectile dysfunction (19.4%)<br>• lack of sexual interest (11.8%)<br>• retarded ejaculation (9.7%)<br>• reduced frequency of masturbation (9.7%) |
| **Jonsson 2003** | ➢ Women 50%<br>➢ Men 75% | • reduced libido<br>• orgasm problems<br>• decreased vaginal lubrication<br>• changes in vaginal sensitivity | • erectile dysfunction<br>• reduced libido |

## 2. Hypothesis

### 2.1. Main Hypothesis

Our main hypothesis was that HD patients experience- in contrast to MS patients- increased and MS patients- in contrast to HD patients- reduced sexual behaviour. This hypothesis was primarily assessed by our own questionnaire titled "Sexuality and partnership in chronic diseases" ("SPCD") as well as by standardised questionnaires (TSST, Sexual functions, FPD, ZIP, FBeK, FLP). In addition there are different supplementary hypotheses that arise from either the hitherto existing literature or from the questionnaires that were used. HD patients experience increased and MS patients reduced sexual behavior.

### 2.2. Supplementary hypotheses

#### 2.2.1. Differences in sexual dysfunction

- MS patients experience sexual dysfunctions.
- HD patients experience sexual dysfunctions.
- **There are significant differences in the sexual dysfunctions between MS and HD patients despite of their similar clinical symptoms** (SPCD, TSST, sexual functions, FLP).

#### 2.2.2. Differences in sexual activities

- HD patients experience hypersexual behaviour.
- MS patients experience hyposexual behaviour.
- **There are significant differences in the sexual activities between patients with MS and those with HD** (SPCD, TSST, Sexual functions, FLP).

#### 2.2.3. Differences in body image and self confidence

- HD patients experience changes in their body image and self confidence.
- HD patients experience changes in their body image and self confidence.
- **There are significant differences in body image and self confidence between patients with MS and those with HD** (FBeK, TSST, PFB).

### 2.2.4. Differences in relationship satisfaction

- HD patients experience difficulties in relationship satisfaction.
- MS patients experience difficulties in relationship satisfaction.
- **There are significant differences in relationship satisfaction between patients with MS and those with HD** (ZIP, sex. function, FLP, PL, TSST, PFB).

## 2.3. Null hypothesis

1. There are no differences in sexual dysfunction between patients with MS and those with HD.
2. There are no differences in relationship satisfaction between patients with MS and those with HD.
3. There are no differences in body image and self confidence between patients with MS and those with HD.

## 3. Patients and Methods
### 3.1. Recruiting of patients
#### 3.1.1. Course of investigations
Patients were first asked by their attending physician if they were willing to take part in the study; afterwards they were approached and informed about the further course of the study. Firstly there was a personal interview of about half an hour where the initiator of the study tried to gather some basic information about the patients' way of life, their partnership and sexual functioning, the duration of the interview depending on the patients' frankness and need to talk about sexuality and pre-existing or illness-accompanying problems. Subsequently the self-report questionnaires were explained to the patients and handed out to them. They completed them either in hospital in the case of inpatients or at home and posted them in the case of outpatients. Some of the Chorea Huntington patients knew the author because of previous group sessions or hospitalisations. The author was completely unknown to all Multiple sclerosis patients. Though, information about the patients' course of disease, their current status and progress of disease was gathered by the authors.

#### 3.1.2. Recruiting of MS patients
Firstly MS outpatients from the MS special ambulance (once a week) Barmherzige Brüder hospital in Graz were recruited over a period of four months. All patients were initially approached by the interviewer while they were waiting in the clinic's waiting room and asked to participate in a survey about sexual problems possibly occurring among MS patients. They were told the study was independent of their treatment in the clinic and any other ongoing research projects.

Secondly, MS patients were recruited from a MS self-help group being shortly introduced to the topic and receiving a lecture about sexuality in MS. Afterwards, all patients were approached by the interviewer and asked to participate in a survey about sexual problems possibly occuring among MS patients. They were informed the study was independent of their treatment in the clinic and any other ongoing research projects.

Thirdly, patients were recruited from a medical specialist for neurology and psychiatry by dispatching written information about the study and asking them to call the interviewer if they were interested to participate in a survey about sexual problems possibly occurring among MS patients. They were informed the study was carried out independently from their treatment at the medical specialist and any other ongoing research projects.

### 3.1.3. Recruiting of HD patients

HD patients were in- and outpatients of the university clinic in Graz at the department of psychiatry. All patients were initially approached by the interviewer and asked to participate in a survey about sexual problems possibly occurring among HD patients. They were told the study was independent of their treatment in the clinic and any other ongoing research projects.

### 3.1.4. Exclusion criteria

Patients were excluded if they
- were unwilling to participate
- were already unable to talk
- suffered from any kind of severe dementia (MMSE<20)

## 3.2. Questionnaires and Problems

There were several difficulties in the investigation of sexual anamnesis in patients which I was also confronted with. The first problem concerning the pre-existing questionnaires was that most of them are in English and just a few of them had been translated into German. Furthermore, most of them require answers from the patients' partners or at least imply that there is a partner which did not hold true for many of the interviewees. On the one hand, some of the forms are very complicated and detailed and could not be used for our patients. On the other hand, some aim at measuring the therapeutic outcome of sexual therapy. In addition, the cooperation with some institutes was difficult so that we never could get hold of some of the questionnaires we had ordered despite of repeated efforts. I have listed the questionnaires taken into consideration below; the ones selected for our study are marked and will be described in detail lateron.

- AHLERS, CJ., GOECKER, D., BEIER, KM. (2001). SFCE SEXUALMEDIZINISCHER FRAGEBOGEN BEI CHRONISCHEN ERKRANKUNGEN
- AHLERS, CJ., SCHAEFER, GA., BEIER, KM. (2002). FSEV FRAGEBOGEN ZUM SEXUELLEN ERLEBEN UND VERHALTEN
- ARENTEWICZ, G., BULLA, R., SCHOOF-TAMS, K., SCHORSCH, E. (1975). FzSV FRAGEBOGEN ZUM SEXUELLEN VERHALTEN
- ARENTEWICZ, G., BULLA, R., SCHOOF-TAMS, K., SCHORSCH, E. (1975). EZS FRAGEBOGEN ZU EINSTELLUNGEN ZUR SEXUALITÄT

- BEIER, KM., AHLERS, CJ., MUNDT, IA., LOEWIT, KK. (2002). 3D INVENTAR ZU DIMENSIONEN VON SEXUALITÄT
- BERNER, MM., KRISTON, L., ZAHRADNIK, H.-P. , HÄRTER, M. & ROHDE, A. (2004). FSFI-D DEUTSCHER FEMALE SEXUAL FUNCTION INDEX
- BÜSING, S., HOPPE, C., LIEDTKE, R. (1997). SEXZUF FRAGEBOGEN SEXUELLE ZUFRIEDENHEIT VON FRAUEN
- CHRISTMANN, F. AND HOYNDORF, S. (1988). FSZ FRAGEBOGEN ZUR SEXUELLEN ZUFRIEDENHEIT
- CROMBACH-SEEBER, B. AND CROMBACH, G. (1977). SII SEXUAL INTERACTION INVENTORY - FRAGEBOGEN ZUR SEXUELLEN INTERAKTION
- ENGFER, A. (1978). PASE PARTNERSCHAFTSFRAGEBOGEN ZUR SEXUALITÄT
- **HAHLWEG, K. (1996). FPD-FLP FRAGEN ZUR LEBENSGESCHICHTE UND PARTNERSCHAFT**
- HARBISON JJM., GRAHAM, PJ., QUINN, JT., MCALLISTER, H., WOODWARD, R. (1977). FRAGEBOGEN ZUR MESSUNG DES SEXUELLEN INTERESSES
- **HASSEBRAUCK, M. (1991). ZIP ZUFRIEDENHEIT IN PAARBEZIEHUNGEN - DEUTSCHE FASSUNG DER RELATIONSHIP ASSESSMENT SCALE VON HENDRICK**
- KLINGLER, OJ. AND LOEWIT, KK. (1996). RSP FRAGEBOGEN "RESSOURCEN IN SEXUALITÄT UND PARTNERSCHAFT"
- LANGER, D. AND LANGER, S. (1988). SFB-F SEXUALFRAGEBOGEN FÜR FRAUEN
- PHILIPPSOHN, S. (2001). F-DSZ FRAGEBOGEN ZU DEN DETERMINANTEN SEXUELLER ZUFRIEDENHEIT
- **STRAUß, B. AND RICHTER-APPELT, H. (1996). FBeK FRAGEBOGEN ZUR BEURTEILUNG DES EIGENEN KÖRPERS.**
- ZIMMER, D. (1989). ASP ANAMNESEBOGEN ZUR SEXUALITÄT UND PARTNERSCHAFT
- ZIMMER, D. (1989). NSP NACHBEFRAGUNGSBOGEN ZUR SEXUALITÄT UND PARTNERSCHAFT
- **ZIMMER, D. (1989). TSST TÜBINGER SKALEN ZUR SEXUALTHERAPIE**

With the selected standardised questionnaires we tried to cover the most important sexual issues as described in literature. In addititon, I made up "my own questionnaire" (called "Sexuality and partnership in chronic diseases"- "SPCD") which in fact was the guideline for the interviews with the patients, covering special questions concerning hypothesis and the most important questions. In the personal interview -being the first part of the study- I divided the answers into four possible groups, namely "Yes"/"No"/"Nor"/"No answer", in order to make it possible to evaluate also this "interviewed questionnaire" to a greater or lesser extend.

I also tried to consider the conditions for negotiation and sexual anamnesis as described by Kockott and Fahrner 2004 (Kockott and Fahrner, 2004).

1. Setting time and space without time pressure and uninterruptedly
2. Influencing the atmosphere of talk by conscious word choice
3. Realising the importance of possible sexual problems
4. Checking the interviewer's own attitude towards sexuality and being aware of possible influences
5. Avoiding moralization and judging of statements from the patients
6. Avoiding only deficit-related questioning by respecting intact areas of sexuality
7. Being conscious of eroticism
8. Approaching the issue slowly if the patients has constraints to talk about sexuality

### 3.2.1. Standardized questionnaires

#### 3.2.1.1. The „Questionnaire for the assessment of spousal relationships" Fragebogen zur Partnerschaftsdiagnostik, FPD (Hahlweg, 1996) consisting of 3 instruments

a) The partnership questionnaire (**PFB** or "Partnerschaftsfragebogen") - specifies partnership quality as consisting of 30 items plus one item for the estimation of happiness. Data for the three scales can be assessed, namely "conflict- behaviour" (items 1, 6, 8, 17, 18, 21, 22, 24, 26, 30), „tenderness"(items 2, 3, 4, 5, 9, 13, 14, 23, 27, 28) and „community/ communication" (items 7, 10, 11, 12, 15, 16, 19, 20, 25, 29). The particular range of each item (1= never to 3= very often) is added to a scalesum (0 to 30). In addition, a total value can be obtained by doing some calculations [(30-scale 1) + scale 2+ scale 3]

b) The list of problems (**PL** or "Problemliste") covers conflictive subjects in partnerships. Answers from 0 ("No conflicts") to 3 ("There are conflicts, but we don't talk about them") are possible. Items with 2 or 3 are also chosen and counted.

c) The questionnaire on life and partnership (**FLP or** "Fragebogen zur Lebensgeschichte und Partnerschaft") gathers further anamnesis information. There is no predetermined analysis for this questionnaire, because it acts as orientation about the current status of the patient's partnership and sexuality. Furthermore, a few questions aimed at collecting some general information about the patient as listed in the following:

1. gender
2. age
5. graduation
9. marital status
13. number of children
16. drugs
18. psychic symptoms
19. marriage of the parents
28. satisfaction with partnership
41. patients attitute in conflicts
50. satisfying sex life
53. orgasm
54. "real" frequency of intercourse
55. desired frequency of intercourse

*3.2.1.2. The „Relationship assessment scale" (RAS)*
*(Zufriedenheit in der Paarbeziehung; ZIP) (Hassebrauck, 1991)*

This scale is a seven-item generic measure of relationship satisfaction. On the scale measurements for love, sexual attitudes, self-disclosure, commitment and investment can be found. This measuring is not limited to marriage relationships and has shown strong predictive validity with dating couples (Vaughn and Baier, 1999). In order to guarantee better comparison in our study we changed the predetermined five ary scale into a six ary scale (1= bad to 6= very good) because all the other used standardised questionnaires have six ary scales, as previously done by Gütl et al. (Gütl et al., 2002).

### Table 6: General data of ZIP

| item | m | SD | s |
|---|---|---|---|
| 1 | 2.32 | .99 | 1.42 |
| 2 | 2.15 | 1.17 | 2.15 |
| 3 | 1.99 | 1.03 | 1.97 |
| <u>4</u> | 2.24 | 1.59 | 2.23 |
| 5 | 2.51 | 1.39 | 1.03 |
| 6 | 1.60 | .82 | 1.17 |
| <u>7</u> | 3.73 | 1.54 | .43 |

m...mean, SD...standard deviation; s...skewness; _ the underlined items had to be pole changed

*3.2.1.3. Questionnaire on self-perception of the body ("Fragebogen zur Beurteilung des eigenen Körpers" or FBeK (Strauß and Richter-Appelt, 1996)*

This is one of the most widespread questionnaires applied in the German-speaking area for assessing peoples' subjective views of their own bodies. The questionnaire consists of 52 items and constitutes a renowned measure of body perception comprising three dimensions, namely attractiveness and self-confidence, insecurity and discomfort, and accentuation of the body and sensitivity (see Table 7). Acceptance or denial of a statement can be expressed by "agree" or "do not agree". Objectivity, reliability and validity are documented and the questionnaire was standardised in 1996 by a sample of 2047 probands.

**Table 7: FBeK**

| Factor 1<br>Insecurity and discomfort | -describing sexual dissatisfaction and paresthesia, lacking feelings and refusal of appearance<br>(19 items- 1, 3, 5, 7, 10, 13, 15, 18, 20, 24, 26, 29, 32, 38, 40, 43, 45, 50, 52) |
|---|---|
| Factor 2<br>Attractiveness and self-confidence | -describing satisfaction with and the image of the own body, attractivity and pleasure in preoccupation with the own body<br>(13 items- 4, 8, 12, 17, 22, 27, 31, 34, 36, 41, 46, 48, 51) |
| Factor 3<br>Accentuation of the body/sensitivity | -describing the feeling of appearance in front of others, mistrust of physical symptoms, concern about health and appearance<br>(20 items- 2, 6, 9, 11, 14, 16, 19, 21, 23, 25, 28, 30, 33, 35, 37, 39, 42, 44, 47, 49) |

_ the underlined items have to be pole changed

## Table 8: General data of FBeK (3-scales)

| scale | m | SD | rit | r | Cα | rtt |
|---|---|---|---|---|---|---|
| Insecurity and discomfort | 5.32 | 4.03 | .40 | .19 | .82 | .67 |
| Attractiveness and self-confidence | 8.91 | 2.91 | .42 | .18 | .75 | .84 |
| Accentuation of the body/ sensitivity | 11.11 | 3.77 | .30 | .12 | .74 | .69 |
| m..mean; SD...Standard deviation; rit...medial discriminatory power; r...medial itemcorrelation; Cα... Cronbachs alpha; rtt...retest reliability ||||||| 

In addition we included the 4-factor re-analysis in our study which is a revised form of the three-scale model. Factor 1 (4) is nearly identical with factor 2 ("attractiveness and self-confidence") and describes satisfaction with one's own body and is also named as the former factor 2. Factor 2 (4) describes one aspect of the former factor 3 ("accentuation of the body/ sensitivity") the accentuation of appearance and pleasure in preoccupation with the own body . Factor 3 (4) "insecurity/ concern" focusses on most of the other items of former factor 3 i.e. the hypochondric view and mistrust of of one's own body and concerns about health. Factor 4(4) "physical-sexual discomfort" describes some items of factor 1 with a focus on sexual problems as well as aspects of shame.

### 3.2.1.4. Tübingen Scales for Sexual Therapy ("Tübinger Skalen zur Sexual-Therapie" or TSST) (Zimmer, 1989)

This scale includes items of different aspects of sexual experience or behaviour and partnership. It can also be used to measure progress in therapeutic processes. On the basis of data analysis of 151 persons there are six factors:

a. Extension of sexual dysfunction
b. Distribution of influence
c. Masturbation
d. Regard and respect
e. Body perception and disgust
f. Communicative fears

There are some problems and points of debate because of the varying spectrum of different items. Most of them are evaluated on a six ary scale (1= "very positive sexual experience" to 6= "very negative sexual experience"). For some items there are scales that have to be more or less transformed by certain defined formulas as follows.

1. For items 1 (frequency of intercourse) and 2 (frequency of masturbation) there is an eight ary scale (1= "never" to 8= "more than five times a week").
Transformation of the raw score:
  1 2 3 4 5 6 7 8 (Raw score)
  6 5 4 3 2 1 1 1 (transformed data)- frequency from 2 or 3 times a week is equated

2. For item 21 (satisfaction after masturbation) and 22 (satisfaction after sexual activity with the partner) there is a possible answer from 0% (never satisfied) to 100% (always satisfied).
Transformation of the percentage (x) into a scale from 1 to 6:
  $[(100-x)/20]+1$

3. Items 22-28 and 35 (extend of arousal/ intensity of orgasm) have positively poled values that have to be transformed:
  $7-x$

4. Item 31 (Distribution of influence in the partnership): from -2 ("the partner has always more influence on decisions") to +2 ("I have always more influence"). This item is divided into 31 a and

b. 31a accumulates all values of the first eleven questions, while 31b accumulates the last 2 questions.

Transformation as follows:

-3   -2   -1        0   +1   +2   +3   (raw scores)- scores more than +3 or less than -3 are assigned to 6

6   5   3   1   2   4   6 (transformed data)

*Calculation of the 6 factors:*

Every item with the same given factor is added up after a transformation that is possibly required and subsequently divided by the number of respective items.

*Factor 1:* 7 items (3, 4, 5, 6, 7, 22 and 29)

*Factor 2:* 5 items (1, 24, 31a, 31b, 35)

*Factor 3:* 4 items (2, 21, 25 and 26)

*Factor 4:* 4 items (20, 32, 33 and 34)

*Factor 5:* 8 items (12, 13, 14, 15, 16, 17, 18 and 19)

*Factor 6:* 3 items (8, 9 and 10)

Items 11, 23, 27, 28 and 30 have no factor and are not integrated into the calculation

#### 3.2.1.5. Sexual Functions (Schulze und Böhm 1990 according to the symptoms' classification by Arentewicz und Schmidt 1986)

The eight items were transformed into a six-ary form, as previously done by Gütl et al. (2002), whereby only item five was left on a three ary scale. The first question was designed to find out if the patients had had sexual intercourse lately. The other items deal with sexual aversion, dysfunction of arousal, dyspareunia, vaginism, anorgasm, orgasm problems, physical and psychic strain. The medial discriminatory power ranges from .13 to .64, the interior consistency is .76.

### 3.2.2. The personal interview

**Sexuality and Partnership in chronic diseases- "SPCD"**

For every question the percentage of possible answers (1= Yes, 2= No, 3= Nor, 4=No answer) was counted. Questions 7b/c, 9b/c, 12b and 14b are only evaluated if answer a) was 1=Yes. Items 7c, 14b and 16 are open questions, possible same answers were counted. For questions a) to e) the average was calculated.

# 4. General data and analysis
## 4.1. General problems

There were some general problems that should at least be mentioned as they add some additional bias to the analysis of this study. As I started with the interviews I was just a medical student in the last part of my studies, but did not have much experience in exploring sexuality in patients. Shortly afterwards, I began to work at the department of psychiatry. With the growing number of patients I had to deal with I learned to cope with these issues, at the end of my studies being much more experienced in carrying out interviews than at the beginning. Nevertheless, many of the patients showed confidence during the interviews and thus talked very frankly about their sexual life and problems. I had many very emotional conversations, not rarely including desperation and teariness. On the other hand, I could also feel the patients' relief to talk about this topic that is often treated as a taboo. The results of this study can never completely reflect all the findings of the interviews as many of them were too personal to be included. Moreover, some patients expressed the wish not to publish everything they told me, which I naturally respected fully.

Furthermore, some problems were encountered in completing the questionnaires. It was my intention that the patients should complete the standardised questionnaires on their own in order to have an additional instrument, being independent from the personal interviews. Unfortunately though, some of the forms returned incompletely, which gave rise to problems in the analysis.

## 4.2. Sociodemografic data

We interviewed 30 HD (1 therefrom excluded) patients and 27 MS patients with the mean age of 42 (42.83 if excluded) (HD) and 43 (MS) years. HD patients were between 24 and 67, MS patients between 28 and 67 years old. 10 HD and 18 MS patients were female, 19 HD and just 9 MS patients were male. All the patients were interviewed personally. 85.19% of the MS patients had a partner while just 66.67% of the HD patients lived in a partnership. 1 female HD patient was interviewed and then excluded because of fullfilling the exclusion criteria (MMSE<22).

If patients had no partner they were only asked to complete the FBeK, if they had a breakup just lately they were also allowed to fill out the other questionnaires by reminding their recent partnership, if they wanted to. The **FBeK** and **ZIP** were completed by 13 HD patients- whereof 2 females and 12 males- and 22 MS patients –whereof 14 were female and 8 male. The **TSST** was filled out by 15 HD patients- 3 females and 12 males- and 22 MS patients (14 females and 8 males), the **FLP** by the aforementioned 22 MS patients and by 17 HD patients(4 female, 13 male). The **PFB** was only completed by 10 HD patients (2 female) but 21 MS patients (14 female and 7 male).

The "**Sexual Functions**" was filled out by 12 HD (2 female) and 21 MS patients (14 female and 7 male).

## 4.3. The interview questionnaire „SPCD"

### 4.3.1.1. Soziodemografic data

The Majority of the MS patients had a partner (85.19%) while just 72.41% of the HD patients lived in a partnership whereof 19 MS (70.37%) and 18 HD (62.07%) patients in a marriage. Just 2 (7.41%) of the MS patients but 6 (20.69%) of the HD patients had been divorced.

37.93% of the HD patients had experienced at least one breakup since the beginning of their illness and 24.14% had begun a new partnership in the meantime, while considerably fewer MS patients had experienced these happenings (breakup: 22.22% , new partner:11.11%) (see table 9).

| Table 9: SPCD | MS (in %) | HD (in%) |
|---|---|---|
| Number of patients | 27 patients | 30 patients |
| Age | 43.04 years | 42.83 years |
| F* | 66.67 | 34.48 |
| m | 33.33 | 67.86 |
| partner | 85.19 | 72.41 |
| divorced | 7.41 | 20.69 |
| married | 70.37 | 62.07 |
| Depression | 62,96 | 58.62 |
| Difficult sex talk | 3.70 | 10.34 |
| Increased sex | 37.04 | 27.59 |
| Decreased sex | 33.33 | 27.59 |
| breakup | 22.22 | 37.93 |
| Partner help | 62.96 | 44.83 |
| jealousy | 40.74 | 10.34 |
| aggression | 55.55 | 44.83 |
| Sexual problems | 59.26 | 20.69 |
| Sex as molestation | 14.81 | 3.45 |
|  | (n.a. 25.93) | (n.a. 44.83) |
| New partner | 11.11 | 24.14 |
| changes | 88.89 | 65.52 |
| Friends help | 59.26 | 58.62 |

n.a.: no answer

*4.3.1.2.Duration and severity of illness*

The mean CAG triplets of all the interviewed HD patients was 46.15 (n=26); the patient with the lowest CAG triplets had 41, the highest 55 repetations. From three patients the result of the genetic testing was not known to us. HD was diagnosed on average 2.64 years ago (n=27), from two patients no data could be obtained. There was a mean onset of disease of 3.46 years (n=22) in the HD patients, from 7 patients no exact data was available (see Table 10).

MS patients had a mean duration of illness of 11.8 years (n=25), only from two patients no data could be available. The exact time of diagnosis was not obtained from most of the MS patients and is therefore not included in the analysis. The mean EDSS of all interviewed patients was 2.87 points; variating between 0 to 7.5 points.

**Table 10 : Mean values of duration and severity of illness**

|  | MS (number of patients) | HD (number of patients) |
|---|---|---|
| **Duration of illness (in years)** | 11.8 (25) | **2.64 (27)** |
| **Onset of disease (in years)** |  | 3.46 (22) |
| **Severity of disease** | 2.87 EDSS (27) | 46.15 CAG (26) |

*4.3.2. "SPCD" analysis*

58.62% of the HD and 62.96% of the MS patients admitted to have depressive episodes but we did not precisely evaluate exact dose or durability as our study more focussed on a cross section of sexuality and partnership- not on the influence of psychopharmacological drugs- in these patients. A detailed list of at present taken medicaments is listed at the FLP results (see Table 16). Interestingly 37.04% (10) MS and 27.59% (8) HD patients reported on sometimes increased sexual interests and activity. Only 9 MS (33.33%) and 8 (27.59%) HD patients reported that they had experienced decreased sexual activity. Reasons for increased and decreased sexual activity as stated by the MS patients are listed in Table 11. A significant higher number of MS patients admitted to have sexual problems (59.26% versus 20.69% HD patients) and to experience sexual activity as molestation (14.81% versus 3.45%). In this context it has to be noted that nearly half of the HD and a quarter of the MS patients did not want to respond to this question. The reported sexual problems are listed below in Table 12.

In addition there is an intersting point concerning the support during their illness. 62.96% of the MS patients indicated that the partner supported them but only 44.83% of the HD patients felt supported by them. Also just 65.52% HD but 88.89% MS patients told that the illness has changed their life. But not only negative changes were reported (see Table 14), many patients of both groups declared to experience also positive consequences, most of them in beeing able to overlook nonrelevant problems and to try to enjoy more every instant of their lifes (see Table 13).

**Table 11: Reasons for sexual changes**

| Reasons for increased sexual interests in MS patients: | Reasons for decreased sexual interests in MS patients: |
|---|---|
| Cortisone (3) | Menopause (2) |
| Associated with menstruation (1) | Cumarine (1) |
| Before reducing Cumarine-therapy (1) | Cortisone (1) |
| Interferon (1) | |

**Table 12: Common problems in sexuality**

| | MS (number of patients) | HD (number of patients) |
|---|---|---|
| Problems to reach orgasm | 6<br>arousal problems (1)<br>extended orgasm (1) | 1 |
| Decreased libido | 4<br>(before/ after acute episode) | 3 |
| Bladderdysfunction (-incontinence, blockade, problems with emptying) | 3 | |
| Erectile dysfunction | 2 | 2 |
| paresthesia | 2 | |
| dry vagina | 1 | |
| Rigidity | 1 | |
| fatigue | 1 | |
| Pain while intercourse | | 1 |

**Table 13: Positive changes**

| Positive changes because of illness (number of patients) | MS | HD |
|---|---|---|
| Try to enjoy life more "carpe diem" | 3 | 6 |
| Closer to family | 2 | 4 |
| Closer to friends | 0 | 2 |
| To wind down, be calm | 1 | 2 |
| Try to take better care of myself | 1 | 1 |
| Be more selfconfident/ respectful | 1 | 1 |
| Works less | 3 | 0 |
| Early retired | 2 | 0 |

**Table 14: Negative changes**

| Negative changes because of illness (number of patients) | MS | HD |
|---|---|---|
| Abandon (Sport, activities..) | 4 | 0 |
| Job-related problems | 3 | 2 |
| Worsening of partnership | 2 | 1 |
| Find oneself guilty of the disease | 1 | 1 |
| Less light-hearted | 1 | 0 |
| Fear and depression | 1 | 0 |
| Harder every-day life | 1 | 0 |

## 4.4. Standardised questionnaires

### 4.4.1. FLP

22 MS and 17 HD patients agreed to fill out the FLP, not all completed it. As the FLP ist normally used at the beginning of sexual therapy not all items were used for statistical analysis. Most of the HD patients had attended either the vocational (Realschule/ berufsbildende höhere Schule- 31.82%) or the high school ("Gymnasium"- 27.27%), while most of the MS patients (82,35%) just had gone to secondary school (Hauptschule).

MS patients had a mean of 1.3 children beeing between 4 and 45 years old, HD patients a mean of 1.5 children (between 4 and 40 years). MS patients also indicated that the marriage of their parents seemed to be quite good or good (63.64%) while many HD patients did not answer to this question and 47.05% reminded a good quality of relationship. Their own partnership estimated most of the MS patients as "happy", more than halfpart of the HD patients as "very happy" (see Table 15).

Table 15: Quality of current partnership

|                | MS (n=21) (in %) | HD (n=13) (in %) |
|----------------|------------------|------------------|
| Very miserable | 0                | 7.69             |
| Miserable      | 4.76             | 0                |
| Quite unhappy  | 14.29            | 0                |
| Rather happy   | 19.05            | 15.38            |
| Happy          | 42.86            | 23.08            |
| Very happy     | 19.05            | 53.85            |

*4.4.1.1.Common physical problems*

The most common physical problems in both groups were difficulties with concentration (22.73% MS, 29.41% HD) and depression (22.73% MS, 23.53% HD). MS patients experienced to a greater extend headache (45.45% MS versus 11.76% HD), inferiority feelings (22.73% MD versus 5.88% HD), Anger (27.27% MS versus 11.76% HD), fear (22.73% MS versus 5.88% HD) and MS patients marked much more often sexual problems as common (27.27% MS versus 5.88% HD).

*4.4.1.2.Drug intake*

In each group 12 patients were taking drugs (MS 54.55%, HD 70.59%). 4 of the MS patients and 2 HD patient were treated with SSRI's (Serotonin reuptake inhibitors), 1 HD patient with trizyclic antidepressives, 1 MS patient with Trazadon, 4 HD patients with Velafaxine and 3 with Mirtazapine, 1 HD patient with flupentixol and 1 with benzodiazepines (see Table 16). 1 MS and 6 HD were treated with atypical neuroleptics, 2 HD were treated with other neuroleptics. For MS specific therapy were 3 MS patients treated with Glatirameracetat, 4 with Interferon and nobody at present with cortisone. 6 MS and 9 HD patients had taken other kinds of drugs.

**Table 16: Actual drug intake**

|  | MS (n=22) (in %) | HD (n=17) (in %) |
|---|---|---|
| Any kind of drug | 54.55 | 70.59 |
| SSRI's | 18.18 | 11.76 |
| Trizyclic antidepressives | 4.55 | 5.88 |
| Trazadone | 4.55 | 0 |
| Venlafaxine | 0 | 23.53 |
| Mirtazapine | 0 | 17.65 |
| Flupentixole | 0 | 5.88 |
| Benzodiazepines | 0 | 5.88 |
| Atypical neuroleptics | 4.55 | 35.29 |
| Other neuroleptics | 0 | 11.76% |
| Other drugs | 27.27 | 52.94 |
|  |  |  |
| Glatirameracetat | 13.64 |  |
| Interferon | 18.18 |  |
| Cortisone | 0 |  |

*4.4.1.3. Frequency of orgasm*

Half of the HD patients indicated to always, the bigger part of the MS patients (47.62%) in the majority of cases to reach orgasm while intercourse, in each group one patient admittet to never orgasm.

*4.4.1.4. Real frequency of intercourse*

26.09% of MS but 40% of HD patients had sex more than once a week, the same percentage of MS and 20% of HD patients indicated sexual activities once a week and 30.44% of MS patients and no HD patient had sex but less than that. 20% of HD and 8.70% of MS patients reported on no sexual activity.

*4.4.1.5. Sexual satisfaction and desired frequency of intercourse*

Most of the patients of both groups declared to be satisfied with their sexual life. The desired frequency of intercourse was high, 38.10% of the MS and 72.73% of the HD patients wished to have intercourse two to three times a week! In addition 14.29% of the MS patients wished to have sex more than three times a week. Furthermore it has to be noted that only 11 patients (64.71%) of the HD patients answered this question.

#### 4.4.1.6. Correlation between "real" and desired frequency of intercourse and orgasm

There was a significant positive correlation between "real" and desired frequency of intercourse and desired frequency of intercourse and orgasm in both groups (see Table 17 and 18).

In HD patients there was significant positive correlation between "real" frequency of sexual intercourse and orgasm which gives evidence that a higher frequency increases the probability of having an orgasm for these patients.

**Table 17: Pearson correlation in HD**

|  | desired frequency of intercourse | "real" frequency of intercourse | Orgasm |
|---|---|---|---|
| **desired frequency of intercourse** | 1 | .864** | .665* |
| "real" frequency of intercourse | .864** | 1 | .654* |
| Orgasm | .665* | .654** | 1 |

* correlation is significant at the 0.05 level (2-tailed)
**correlation is significant at the 0.01 level (2-tailed)

**Table 18: Pearson correlation in MS**

|  | desired frequency of intercourse | "real" frequency of intercourse | Orgasm |
|---|---|---|---|
| **desired frequency of intercourse** | 1 | .734** | .475* |
| "real" frequency of intercourse | .734** | 1 | .377 |
| Orgasm | .475* | .377 | 1 |

* correlation is significant at the 0.05 level (2-tailed)
**correlation is significant at the 0.01 level (2-tailed)

### 4.4.2. TSST

In the TSST higher values refer to problems, lower values to satisfaction in the particular item. Statistical analysis can be obtained from table 19 and 20. The MS patients showed significant higher rates in the extend of sexual dysfunction of factor 1, which includes problems of the whole sexual circle and the general satisfaction with sexual intercourse (see table 19). In addition they experienced a significant lower intensity of sexual arousal, had a lower frequency of intercourse and a lower influence on sexual initiative in comparison to HD patients (factor 2). These, in contrast, feel more attractive and respected in their partnership (factor 4) and commit less fear from an active role in sexuality and expression of own wishes (factor 6). There were no significant differences in intensity and frequency of masturbation (factor 3), disgust of male or female bodysecrets or image of the own body or the partner (factor 5). In this context it has to be mentioned that especially the issue of masturbation was just completed entirely by 50% of the HD and <2/3 of the MS patients and apparently remains a taboo-subject as also previous shown by Gütl et al. (2002).

Interestingly mean values of HD patients in "sexual dysfunction", "influence", "Regard and respect" and "communicative fears" were not increased- sometimes even decreased- in comparison to the mean values of the general population (sexual unstressed men), leading to the assumption of a possibly more uncritical view of sexual issues (see table 19).

**Table 19: TSST Descriptives**

|  | Patients HD (n= 15) MS (n= 22) | mean | sexual burdened men general | Norming sample-men |
|---|---|---|---|---|
| sexual dysfunction* | HD | 1.521 | 3.03 | 1.64 |
|  | MS | 2.181 |  |  |
| Influence* | HD | 1.90 | 3.37 | 2.51 |
|  | MS | 3.07 |  |  |
| Masturbation | HD | 3.96 (n.a. 8) | 4.00 | 2.50 |
|  | MS | 3.50 (n.a.8) |  |  |
| Regard and Respect* | HD | 1.14 | 2.62 | 1.81 |
|  | MS | 1.78 |  |  |
| Body perception and disgust | HD | 2.12 | 2.75 | 2.34 |
|  | MS | 2.32 |  |  |
| Communicative fears* | HD | 1.42 | 3.09 | 1.85 |
|  | MS | 2.17 |  |  |

n.a. (8): 8 patients did not answer to this question;* significant different p<0.05 between MS and HD

Table 20: Analysis of variance (ANOVAs, TSST)

|  | Sum of squares | df | Mean S | F (1,37) | p |
|---|---|---|---|---|---|
| sexual dysfunction* | 4.035 | 1 | 4.035 | 4.457 | 0.042 |
| Influence* | 12.575 | 1 | 12.575 | 8.448 | 0.006 |
| Masturbation | 1.958 | 1 | 1.958 | 0.789 | 0.380 |
| Regard and Respect* | 3.790 | 1 | 3.790 | 6.765 | 0.013 |
| Body perception and disgust | 0.396 | 1 | 0.396 | 0.439 | 0.512 |
| Communicative fears* | 5.211 | 1 | 5.211 | 4.460 | 0.042 |

* significant different p<0.05

### 4.4.3. FBeK 3-scales

We calculated analysis of variance of the 3-scales version after verifying normal distribution (see table 21 and 22). In the FBeK 3-scales version HD patients indicated lower levels of insecurity and discomfort (scale 1). They seem to experience significant higher sexual satisfaction while MS patients experience more negative feelings concerning their body and appearance. In addition they seem to feel less attractive and selfconfident (scale 2) and trust to a significantly lesser extend in their body in comparison to the HD patients (scale 3). It is astonishing that the latter also have significant higher levels than the norming sample in scale 2, which would indicate increased selfconfidence and increased pleasure in preoccupation with the own body. Also in scale 3 HD patients had lower levels, seemingly to be less concerned about their health and less sensitive to their appearance in comparison to the MS patients but also to the norming sample.

Table 21: FBeK 3-scales : Descriptives

|  | patients | Mean value | Norming sample | Confidence interval |
|---|---|---|---|---|
| Scale 1* insecurity and discomfort | HD | 4.41 |  |  |
|  | MS | 8.00 | 5.32 | 4,022 – 6,619 |
| Scale 2* attractiveness and self-confidence | HD | 10.00 |  |  |
|  | MS | 7.91 | 8.91 | 7,972 – 9,848 |
| Scale 3* | HD | 9.82 |  |  |

| accentuation of the body/ sensitivity | MS | 12.68 | 11.11 | 9,895 – 12,32 |

* significant different between HD and MS $p<0.05$

### Table 22: FBeK 3-scales: Analysis of variance

|  | Sum of squares | df | Mean S | F (1,38) | Sig. |
|---|---|---|---|---|---|
| **Scale 1 *** | 123.472 | 1 | 123.472 | 8.396 | 0.006 |
| Scale 2 * | 41.925 | 1 | 41.925 | 5.244 | 0.028 |
| Scale 3 * | 78.844 | 1 | 78.844 | 6.100 | 0.018 |

* significant different $p<0.05$

#### 4.4.4. FBeK 4-scales

In addtition to the 3-scales version of the FBeK analysis of variance of the 4-scales version was calculated, as recommended in the original version of the questionnaire (see table 23 and 24). Scale 1, 3 and 4 were significantly differing in the two patient groups. Only scale 2- displaying the "postive" aspects of the former factor 3- the accentuation of appearance and pleasure in preoccupation with the own body- was not signifcant different. As in the 3-scale version HD patients felt significant more attractive and selfconfident (scale 1), had significant lower levels of insecurity and concern about their body and health (scale 3) and indicated fewer sexual problems and lower levels of shame (scale 4). The results of the 4-scale version of the FBeK confirms more or less the results of the 3-scale version (1=2, 2=3, 3=3, 4=1).

### Table 23: FBeK 4-scales: Descriptives

|  | HD (n=16) | MS (n=22) |
|---|---|---|
| Scale 1* Attractiveness/selfconfidence | 12.18 | 9.59 |
| Scale 2 accentuation of body/ sensitivity | 6.12 | 7.27 |
| Scale 3* insecurity/ concern | 4.59 | 7.59 |

| Scale 4* physical-sexual discomfort | .94 | 2.73 |
|---|---|---|

* significant different p<0.05

**Table 24: FBeK 4-scales: Analysis of variance**

|  | Sum of squares | df | Mean S | F (1,38) | p |
|---|---|---|---|---|---|
| Scale 1* | 64.109 | 1 | 64.109 | 6.054 | 0.019 |
| Scale 2 | 12.795 | 1 | 12.795 | 2.688 | 0.110 |
| Scale 3* | 86.462 | 1 | 86.462 | 9.594 | 0.004 |
| Scale 4* | 30.593 | 1 | 30.593 | 13.269 | 0.001 |

* significant different p<0.05

### 4.4.5. ZIP

We calculated the 2 tailed significance of analysis of variance after discovering that most of the items of the ZIP were not normal distributed (see Table 25). Relationship satisfaction measured by the ZIP arised significant differences in the two patient groups in five of seven questions. HD patients showed significant higher need and partnership satisfaction (item 1 and 2), partnership met significant more their primary expectations and significant more HD patients declared to love their partner than MS patients (item 5 and 6). In addition MS patients indicated to have more problems in their partnership (item 7). There was no significant difference between the groups in how they appreciated their relationship in comparison to others and how often they wished not to be in the actual partnership.

**Table 25: ZIP: analysis of variance**

| | patients | Mean rank | Sum of ranks | Mann-Whitney-U | Sig. (2-tailed) |
|---|---|---|---|---|---|
| Fulfils desire* | HD | 11.88 | 154.50 | 63.5 | 0.004 |
| | MS | 21.61 | 475.50 | | |
| Satisfaction* | HD | 12.42 | 161.50 | 70.5 | 0.008 |
| | MS | 21.30 | 468.50 | | |
| In comparison | HD | 14.27 | 185.50 | 94.5 | 0.091 |
| | MS | 19.50 | 409.50 | | |
| Better not | HD | 14.88 | 193.50 | 102.5 | 0.105 |
| | MS | 19.12 | 401.50 | | |
| Expectations* | HD | 12.50 | 162.50 | 71.5 | 0.015 |
| | MS | 20.60 | 432.50 | | |
| Love* | HD | 13.50 | 175.50 | 84.5 | 0.018 |
| | MS | 20.66 | 454.50 | | |
| Problems* | HD | 11.19 | 145.50 | 54.5 | 0.002 |
| | MS | 22.02 | 484.50 | | |

\* **significant different p<0.05**

### 4.4.6. Sexual Functions

A very high number of both patient groups indicated to have had sexual activity lately (although "lately" is to construe extensively) (see table 26). All of the HD patients had positive feelings before sexual contact (agreeable/ very agreeable/ feel like it) while 14.29% of the MS patients reported to feel disagreeable (table 27). During intercourse one patient of each group had always pain and other problems, just a few patients of each group experienced often pain while intercourse 8.33% of HD and 4.76% of MS patients). Significantly more of the HD patients experienced high or very high levels of arousal at intercourse (83.34%) which was just reported by 38.10% of the MS patients. 91.67% of the HD and 47.62% of the MS patients reported to have had an orgasm lately. Physical and psychical satisfaction (allways and almost allways) was very high in most of the HD patients (91.67%), just 57.15% of the MS patients felt physical and 61.92% psychical satisfied after sexual intercourse (table 28 and 29).

**Table 26: Sex lately**

|           | MS (n=21) (in %) | HD (n=12) (in %) |
|-----------|------------------|------------------|
| Yes       | 66.67            | 81.82            |
| No        | 33.33            | 16.67            |
| No answer | 0                | 8.33             |

**Table 27: Before sexual contact**

|                | MS (n=21) (number of patients) | HD (n=12) (number of patients) |
|----------------|-------------------------------|-------------------------------|
| Feel harassed  | 0     | 0     |
| Disagreeable   | 14.29 | 0     |
| Unconcerned    | 9.53  | 0     |
| Agreeable      | 28.57 | 8.33  |
| Very agreeable | 14.29 | 25.00 |
| Feel like it   | 28.57 | 66.67 |
| No answer      | 4.76  | 0     |

Positiv feelings: HD 100% versus MS 71.43%
Negativ feelings: HD 0% versus MS 14.29%

**Table 28: Physical satisfaction after intercourse**

|        | MS (n=21) (in %) | HD (n=12) (in %) |
|--------|------------------|------------------|
| Never  | 0                | 8.33             |
| Seldom | 9.52             | 0                |

| | | |
|---|---|---|
| Sometimes | 23.81 | 0 |
| Often | 4.76 | 0 |
| Almost always | 33.34 | 25 |
| Always | 23.81 | 66.67 |
| No answer | 4.76 | 0 |

**Table 29: Psychical satisfaction after intercourse**

| | MS (n=21) (in %) | HD (n=12) (in %) |
|---|---|---|
| Never | 9.52 | 8.33 |
| Seldom | 4.76 | 0 |
| Sometimes | 9.52 | 0 |
| Often | 9.52 | 0 |
| Almost always | 14.29 | 16.67 |
| Always | 47.63 | 75 |
| No answer | 4.76 | 0 |

### 4.4.7. PFB

In the "Questionnaire of partnership" MS patients indicated more problems in all three items. That means that they had more difficulties in finding attitudes to dissolve conflicts ("conflict-behavior"), in physical contact ("tenderness") and in common activities with the partner ("community and communication") (see table 30).

**Table 30: Results of PFB**

| | MS (n=21) | HD (n= 10) |
|---|---|---|
| Mean S "conflict-behavior" | 7.0 | 5.1 |
| Mean Z "tenderness" | 18.2 | 23.8 |
| Mean G | 18.0 | 23.6 |

| | | |
|---|---|---|
| „community/ communication" | | |
| Total value | 59.2 | 72.3 |

### 4.4.8. PL

The most prevalent problems in the relationship can be obtained from Table 31. On the whole HD patients indicated significantly fewer problems than MS patients.

**Table 31: List of problems in the partnership**

| | MS (n=19) (number of patients) | HD (n=11) (number of patients) |
|---|---|---|
| 7. Temperament of partner | 21.05 | 0 |
| 11. Jealousy | 10.53 | 9.09 |
| 12. Give personal leeway | 5.26 | 9.09 |
| 13. Sexuality | 21.05 | 0 |
| 15. Relatives | 31.58 | 9.09 |
| 17. Communication | 5.26 | 9.09 |
| 18. Desire to start a family | 5.26 | 9.09 |
| 19. Missing acceptance | 15.79 | 9.09 |
| 20. Demands of the partner | 15.79 | 0 |

## 4.5. Correlations

### 4.5.1. Correlation between TSST, sum of ZIP, FLP, age and duration of illness

Pearson correlation was calculated for all the scales of the TSST that were significant differing in both groups (scale 1, 2, 4 and 6) and correlated with each other as well as with the sum of ZIP, age of patients and duration of illness, desired and real frequency of intercourse and orgasm (see Table 32).

*TSST and Sum of ZIP.* It showed in both groups a significant positive correlation between "regard and respect" (TSST) and "sum of ZIP". That means that the more patients felt attractive and respected by their partner the more they had experienced happiness and satisfaction in their relationship. In addition in HD patients there was a significant positive correlation between "regard and respect" (TSST) and "communicative fears" (TSST) and between "regard and respect" and "influence" (TSST). That means that taking an active role in sexuality and having the heart to express own wishes was directly linked with attractiveness and respect in the partnership. If HD patients had a high level of influence in the partnership as well as high levels of arousal and a high frequency of intercourse they experienced higher feelings of respect and attractiveness in their partnership. A similar result was given by the significant positive correlation between "communicative fears" (TSST) and the "sum of ZIP", less fear of an active role in sexuality and expression of own wishes was linked with high happiness in the partnership.

It is interesting that there was a significant positive correlation between the "sum of ZIP" and "sexual dysfunction" (TSST) only in HD patients but not in MS patients, which means that for MS patients the level of sexual dysfunction and satisfaction is not associated with happiness in their partnership, while for HD patients this is indeed the case in this study.

For MS patients a significant positive relation between "communicative fears" (TSST) and "sexual dysfunction" (TSST) could be shown. They experienced high levels of fear of an active role in sexuality and expression of own wishes which was directly linked to high sexual dysfunction. Consistent with this result there is a significant positive correlation between "Influence" (TSST) and "communicative fears" (TSST) which means that the fear of an active role in sexuality and of the expression of own wishes is linked with a lower intensity of sexual arousal, lower frequency of intercourse and lower influence on sexual initiative.

The significant positive correlation between "influence" (TSST) and "sexual dysfunction" (TSST) is obvious as a lower intensity of sexual arousal, lower frequency of intercourse and lower influence on sexual initiative accords to more sexual dysfunction.

There was no correlation with age or duration of illness in neither of the groups.

*FLP and TSST.* In MS patients a significant negative correlation between "desired frequency of intercourse" and "sexual dysfunction", "influence" and "communicative fears" could be found. In addition there was a significant negative correlation between "real frequency of intercourse" and "sexual dysfunction", "influence" and "communicative fears". This gives evidence that MS patients with more sexual dysfunctions, a lower influence on sexual activity and a very inactive role in sexuality wish to have sexual activities rarely. Furthermore the significant negative correlation between "orgasm" and "sexual dysfunction", "influence" and "communicative fears" shows that patients with more sexual dysfunctions, a lower influence on sexual activity and a very inactive role in sexuality less frequent experience orgasm.

In HD patients there was a significant positive correlation between "desired frequency of intercourse" and "regard and respect" and "communicative fears". At the same time there was a significant positive correlation between real frequency of intercourse and regard and respect and communicative fears. This would mean that HD patients- even if they felt less attractive and respected in their partnership as well if they were not taking an active role in sexuality and didn't have much heart to express own wishes they wished to have a higher frequency of intercourse. These contradictory correlations is to interpret carefully as only 11 patients completed the questionnaires and eight of eleven HD patients indicated to wish to have sex two to three times a week. If results should be interpreted nevertheless this would- in my opinion- show a high level of disihibition despite the low progression of cognitive degradation or patients.

### 4.5.2. Correlation between FBeK, ZIP and SPCD

The three scales of the FBeK were correlated with each other, the sum of ZIP and 5 items of the SPCD ("Increased sexual activity", "decreased sexual activity", "sexual problems", "breakup since illness" and "new partnership since illness").

There was a significant positive correlation for all patients between the three scales of the FBeK. This shows that patients who experience higher sexual dissatisfaction, paresthesia or lacking feelings (scale1) are less satisfied with the image of the own body (scale 2) and are more concerned about their health and appearance (scale 3) and vice versa. There was no correlation between age, "increased" or "decreased sexual activity", "sum of ZIP", "sexual problems", "new partner" or "breakup since the illness".

**Table 32a: Pearson correlation: MS**

| Number of patients: n=21 | Sexual dysfunction (TSST) | Influence (TSST) | Regard & respect (TSST) | Communicative fears (TSST) | Desired frequency (FLP) |
|---|---|---|---|---|---|
| Sexual dysfunction | 1 | .841** | .361 | .839** | -.664** |
| Influence | .841** | 1 | .235 | .704** | -.457* |
| Regard & respect | .361 | .235 | 1 | .311 | -.267 |
| Communicative fear | .839** | .704** | .311 | 1 | -.641** |
| Desired frequency | -.664** | -.475* | -.367 | -.641** | 1 |
| Real frequency | -.663** | -.648** | -.249 | -.661** | .734** |
| Orgasm | -.778** | -.653** | -.335 | -.715** | .475* |
| Sum ZIP (n=20) | .412.412 | .499* | .486* | .310 | -.169 |
| Age | .043 | .078 | .415 | -.010 | .103 |
| Duration of illness (n=20) | .011 | -.029 | .404 | -.069 | -.061 |

*correlation is significant at the 0.05 level (2-tailed); **correlation is significant at the 0.01 level (2-tailed)

**Table 32b: Pearson correlation: MS**

| Number of patients: n=21 | Real frequency (FLP) | Orgasm (FLP) | Sum ZIP | Age | Duration of illness (SPCD) |
|---|---|---|---|---|---|
| Sexual dysfunction | -.663** | -.778** | .412 | .043 | .011 |
| Influence | -.648** | -.653** | .499* | .078 | -.029 |
| Regard and respect | -.249 | -.335 | .486* | .415 | .404 |
| Communicative fears | -.661** | -.715** | .310 | -.010 | -.069 |
| Desired frequency | .734** | .475* | -.169 | .103 | -.061 |
| Real frequency | 1 | .377 | -.435 | .129 | -.017 |
| Orgasm | .377 | 1 | -.344 | -.128 | -.249 |
| Sum ZIP (n=20) | -.435 | -.344 | 1 | .391 | .314 |
| Age | .129 | -.182 | .391 | 1 | .364 |
| Duration of illness (n=20) | -.017 | -.249 | .314 | .364 | 1 |

*correlation is significant at the 0.05 level (2-tailed); **correlation is significant at the 0.01 level (2-tailed)

## 4.6. Case reports
### 4.6.1. HD patients
*4.6.1.1. Case 1*

One male patient, experiencing sexual dysfunctionsince some years, told me his further plans concerning sexuality. He was concerned about the sex life of his wife and her missing sexual satisfaction. He wanted to ask his son-in-law to overtake the sexual part with his wife as her sexual partner. He had already talked to his wife about it but had not thought about the feelings of his daughter or possible reactions of the son-in-law. The HD patient felt confident and proud with his decision and did not waste any thoughts on the feelings of the rest of the family.

*4.6.1.2. Case 2*

One female patient, with whom I performed a personal interview who afterwards had to be excluded from the analysis because of severe dementia, attracted attention while being inpatient. Despite negating sexual increased behaviour in the personal interview she showed uninhibited behavior by entering unknown sickrooms and trying to fondle other male patients by touching their genitals. In addition she was discovered while having sexual intercourse with another patient in the toilet rooms in the hospital.

### 4.6.2. MS patient
*4.6.2.1. Case 1*

One female patient reported in the interview that she recently has had an extended orgasm lasting nearly one day. She was all the time experiencing orgasmic waves without being able to stop it and felt very uncomfortable while this episode. She reported to have much fear that it could happen again and is therefore really afraid of having sexual activities.

# 5. Discussion
## 5.1. Testing of hypotheses
### 5.1.1. Main hypothesis.

For testing of our *main hypothesis*- that HD patients experience in contrast to MS patients increased and MS patients in contrast to HD patients reduced sexual behavior- results of the personal interview SPCD and the standardised questionnaires TSST, sexual functions, PFB, FLP ("number of children", "orgasm", "real frequency of intercourse", "desired frequency of intercourse"), ZIP ("problems in the partnership") and FBeK 3-scales ("attractiveness and self-confidence") have been evaluated.

In the personal interview 33.33% of the MS and 27.59% of the HD patients reported on decreased sexual activity. Interestingly an even slightly higher percetage of MS patients also stated to know increased sexual interest and behavior (37.04% versus 27.59% HD patients), only some of them related to cortisone therapy. A very high number of both patient groups indicated to have had sexual activity lately (66.67% MS versus 81.82% HD patients) (Sexual functions-"Sex lately") but in fact most of the HD patients experienced high or very high levels of arousal at intercourse (83.34%) which was just reported by 38.10% of the MS patients. All HD patients had positive feelings before sexual contact while 14.29% of the MS patients reported to feel disagreeable (Sexual functions-"Sex lately", "Before sexual contact", "Arousal at intercourse "; TSST- "influence"). Half of the HD patients indicated to always, the bigger part of the MS patients in the majority of cases to reach orgasm while intercourse and had less fear from an active role in sexuality and expression of own wishes in contrast to the MS patients (TSST- "communicative fears"). In comparing the groups concerning the real frequency of intercourse about one quarter of MS but 40% of HD patients had sex more than once a week, a similar percentage for both groups indicated sexual activities once a week and 20% HD and twice as many MS patients less than that. HD patients had also a higher desired frequency of intercourse- 72.73% of the HD and 38.10% of the MS patients wished to have intercourse two to three times a week- although only 11 patients (64.71%) of the HD patients answered this question. Interestingly additionally 14.29% of the MS patients wished to have sex more than three times a week (FLP- "orgasm", "real frequency of intervcourse", "desired frequency of intercourse"; TSST- "influence").

The subject of masturbation apparently remains a taboo-subject as nearly half of all patients did not answer to this question. There was no difference in intensity and frequency of masturbation in the answering patients (TSST- "masturbation").

MS patients had a mean of 1.3 children beeing between 4 and 45 years old, HD patients a mean of 1.5 children (between 4 and 40 years). This is a bit lower than the Austrian mean indicating that the

Austrians had a mean of 1.67 (2004) and 1.69 (2005) children per household (Statistik Austria) (FLP- "number of children"). In addition MS patients indicated to have more problems in their partnership and seem to feel less attractive and selfconfident and to trust to a significantly lesser extend in their body in comparison to the HD patients (PFB, ZIP- "problems in the partnership"; TSST- "influence", "communicative fears").

Concurrent with these observations HD patients even indicated fewer problems than the norming sample in different items (FBeK 3-scales- "attractiveness and self-confidence"; TSST- "influence", "communicative fears"). They therewith seem to have increased selfconfidence, to be less concerned about their health and less sensitive to their appearance, to have higher levels of sexual arousal, a higher frequency of intercourse, a higher influence on sexual initiative and less fear from an active role in sexuality and expression of own wishes. This could lead to the assumption of a possibly more uncritical view of sexual issues and therewith confirm our main hypothesis for the HD patients of increased sexual behaviour. For the MS patients the main hypothesis of decreased sexual behavior seems to be approved in most of the items but as more MS than HD patients indicated to know sexual increased behavior and a seventh part of them wished to have sex more than three times a week it gives evidence that also increased sexual activity is prevalent.

### 5.1.2. Supplementary hypothesis

*5.1.2.1. First supplementary hypothesis*

The first supplementary hypothesis that there are significant differences in the sexual dysfunctions between MS and HD patients despite of their similar clinical symptoms has been evaluated by the SPCD, the TSST ("Sexual dysfunction", "influence") the Sexual functions ("Arousal at intercourse", "Orgasm", "Orgasm lately", "Pain at intercourse", "Problems at intercourse", "Orgasm ") and the FLP ("satisfying sex life", "orgasm").

A significant higher number of MS patients admitted to have sexual problems (SPCD, TSST "sexual dysfunction" ) whereof one patient of each group had always pain or other problems during intercourse (Sexual functions- "Pain at intercourse", "Problems at intercourse"). Most of the patients of both groups declared to be satisfied with their sexual life (FLP- "satisfying sex life") only a small number of patients indicated to experience sexual activity as molestation (14.81% MS versus 3.45% HD patients). Most of the HD patients experienced high levels of arousal at intercourse (83.34%) which was just reported by 38.10% of the MS patients (Sexual functions- "Arousal at intercourse"; TSST- "influence"). Half of the HD patients indicated to always, the bigger part of the MS patients in the majority of cases, to reach orgasm while intercourse and nearly all (91.67%) of the HD and 47.62% of the MS patients reported to have had an orgasm lately (sexual functions "orgasm", "orgasm lately"; FLP- "orgasm").

Recapitulatory our results show that MS patients admitted to have more sexual problems, lower levels of arousal and fewer orgasm than HD patients. The most common sexual problems were problems in reaching orgasm, decreased libido and erectile dysfunction in both groups, in addition bladder dysfunction was prevalent in MS patients. Nevertheless sexual activity seems to be satisfying for most of the patients.

*5.1.2.2. Second supplementary hypothesis*

The second supplementary hypothesis that there are significant differences in the sexual activities between patients with MS and those with HD was evaluated by the SPCD, the TSST ("communicative fear", "masturbation"), the Sexual functions ("Sex lately") and the FLP ("desired frequency of intercourse", "real frequency of intercourse").

A very high number of patients indicated to have had sexual activity lately (66.67% MS versus 81.82% HD patients) (Sexual functions-"Sex lately") and there were no significant differences in intensity and frequency of masturbation (TSST- "masturbation"). The results of the TSST resulted in a confirmation of the hyposexual behavior of MS patients as they had more fear from an active role in sexuality and expression of own wishes (TSST- "communicative fears"). A fewer number of HD patients indicated to know increased (27.59% HD versus 37.04% MS patients) or decreased (27.59% HD versus 33.33% MS patients) sexual activity in the personal interview (SPCD). The desired frequency of intercourse was high, 38.10% of the MS and 72.73% of the HD patients wished to have intercourse two to three times a week. In addition 14.29% of the MS patients wished to have sex more than three times a week. Furthermore it has to be noted that only 11 patients (64.71%) of the HD patients answered this question (FLP- "desired frequency of intercourse", "real frequency of intercourse"). These results comfirm the experience of increased sexual behavior of the HD patients only partially and contradict this second supplementary hypothesis in the case of MS patients.

*5.1.2.3. Third supplementary hypothesis*

The third supplementary hypothesis that there are significant differences in body image and self confidence between patients with MS and those with HD was evaluated by the FBeK (3-scales- "attractiveness and self-confidence"; 4-scales- "accentuation of body/ sensitivity", "insecurity/ concern"), the TSST ("body perception and disgust") and the PFB.

HD patients seem to experience significant higher sexual satisfaction while MS patients experience more negative feelings concerning their body and appearance. In addition they seem to feel less attractive and selfconfident while HD patients had significant lower levels of insecurity and concern about their body and health (FBeK 3-scales- "attractiveness and self-confidence"; FBeK 4-scales- "insecurity/ concern", PFB). There were no significant differences in disgust of male or female bodysecrets or image of the own body or the partner and the accentuation of appearance and pleasure in preoccupation with the own body (FBeK 4-scales- "accentuation of body/ sensitivity"; TSST "body perception and disgust"). This leads us to the assumption of increased selfconfidence, higher sexual satisfaction and low concern abouth body and health in HD patients in contrast to MS patients.

### 5.1.2.4. Fourth supplementary hypothesis.

The fourth supplementary hypothesis that there are significant differences in relationship satisfaction between patients with MS and those with HD was evaluated by the SPCD, the TSST ("regard and respect", "communicative fears"), the ZIP (all 7 items), the Sexual functions ("Physical satisfied, "Psychical satisfied"), the PL, the FLP ("satisfaction with partnership") and the PFB.

HD patients experienced significantly more breakups than MS patients and also more of them had begun a new relationship since they were ill (see table). In addition only 44.83% reported to feel supported by their partner while 55.55% of the MS patients felt helped by their partner (SPCD). MS patients indicated to be significantly more jealous and slightly to feel more aggressiv than HD patients (SPCD). The results of the TSST verified that HD patients felt more attractive and respected in their partnership and had less fear from an active role in sexuality and expression of own wishes in contrast to the MS patients but also to the norming sample (TSST- "regard and respect", "communicative fears").

HD patients showed higher need and partnership satisfaction, their partner met significantly more their primary expectations and significant more HD patients declared to love their partner than MS patients and to have fewer problems in their partnership (ZIP; FLP- "satisfaction with partnership", PFB, PL). Physical and psychical satisfaction was very high in most of the HD patients (91.67%) while just 57.15% of the MS patients felt physical and 61.92% psychical satisfied after sexual intercourse (Sexual functions- "Physical satisfied, "Psychical satisfied").

These results confirm this fourth supplementary hypothesis that there are significant differences in partnership satisfaction as MS patients experience lower levels and HD patients partly even higher levels than the norming sample. It has to be said that nevertheless HD patients experienced more breakups than MS patients leading to the assumption of a noncritical view of relationship in HD.

## 5.2. Interpretation

How can these results now be explained? The first question arising is the one of a possibly high social desirability, which has not been evaluated, especially in HD. Nearly all of them indicated to be perfect lovers and partners, having only a few problems by feeling very self-confident and attractive. About 30% reported on previous increased sexual activities- which concurs with the literature (Fedoroff et al., 1994)- the same percentage on decreased sexual interests, concerning this matter the hitherto literature is differing between less than 10% to over 70% (Fedoroff et al., 1994, Craufurd et al., 2001). Considering the severity and progression of the disease, with all the omnipresent problems for the patients themselves but also their families, it is astonishing with what courage to face their life most of the patients- at least reported to- cope with their destiny. HD patients did not report on increased but decreased real sexual frequency, but indicated indirectly increased sexual desire and uncritical views of sexuality and partnership. Does this also refer to hypersexuality?

In addition the bigger part of HD patients was taking any kind of drugs, significantly more HD than MS patients were taking psychotropics. This would allow the assumption of induced sexual problems which were though not reported. For further verification of data, it would have been necessary to interview partners or other family members which has not been possible for this study.

MS patients indeed seem to face their illness more realistically, but also here it is astonishing that most of the patients reported to be satisfied with their sex life despite various sexual problems. Relationships seem- in addition- to be more stable than in HD disease in spite of reduced self-confidence and lower subjective initiative on sexual activities. Partnership happiness and duration of illness was not directly correlated with sexual satisfaction in MS This could confirm the results from the literature were the majority of MS patients experienced high levels of sexual dysfunctions but was not concerned or was only a bit concerned about the sexual difficulties (McCabe et al., 1996). Possibly MS patients are more able to find an alternative interpersonal level with their partners despite sexual dysfunctions and reduced libido. In addition hypersexuality, sometimes but not always related to cortisone therapy- seems to be prevalent. As reported in our case report- possibly spastic and abnormal muscle regulation can cause rare and extraordinary genital symptoms as extended orgasm.

Furthermore the disinhibited attitutes of HD patients and the very outstanding behavior of the two reported HD cases cause considerations. One theory explaining the present results could in both groups be the disappearance of inhibitions which is though discussed in advanced stages and related to dementia which does not apply to our patient groups. Possibly incipient development-especially in HD- is responsible for the unwounded view and easy taking behavior. This had also been obvious in the personal interviews where I often had been confronted with tears and severe desperation of MS patients while nearly all of the HD patients remained factual and inapproachable often seeming not to be aware of their problems.

The significant differences in the sexual and partnership behavior between MS and HD patients- despite that all of them experienced the social consequences of their disease- leads to the conclusion that the both patient groups seem to cope with their illness in a totally different way. In addition the underlying organic changes seem to have a great impact on personality structur and behavior. From a psychodynamical point of view the role of the disinhibited behavior and outstanding symptoms seems to be interesting in HD. Psychodynamic theories assume that each disease covers deeper conflicts and the way it is managed represents the creative fight of life to survive. In the illness the psychodynamic of ones life, the relation to oneself and to the environment becomes obvious. In addition in some aspects the disease is created and needed and used to modulate the social environment (Pieringer, 2007). In HD outweighing an extraordinary illness by an extraordinary behavior could be assumed.

# 6. Conclusion

About one third of the patients of both groups reported on sometimes decreased sexual activity, an even slightly higher percetage of MS patients also stated to know increased sexual interest and behavior, only some of them related to cortisone therapy. In comparing the groups concerning the real frequency of intercourse about one quarter of MS but 40% of HD patients had sex more than once a week seeming to have decreased sexual activities also in contrast to the normal population in Europe where 60% of men and 56% of women between 40 and 49 years had sex more than once a week (Nicolosi et al., 2006). But contradictory in most of the other items HD patients indicated increased sexual interest and higher levels of arousal, less negative feelings before and after sexual contact and more frequent orgasm. In the partnership they had less fear from an active role in sexuality and expression of own wishes and to have less problems in their partnership in contrast to the MS patients. The last-mentioned indicated to feel less attractive and self-confident and to trust to a significantly lesser extend in their body in comparison to the HD patients. Concurrent with these observations HD patients even indicated fewer problems than the norming sample in different items. This leads us to the assumption of a possibly more uncritical view of sexual issues in HD but also gives evidence that increased sexual activity is prevalent in MS although problems in sexuality and partnership seem to be more frequent. In addition HD patients experienced more break-ups of relationship than MS patients despite significant higher satisfaction leading to the supposition of a transfigured view in HD. As distinctive feature concerning sexuality in still asymptomatic patients it would be interesting to know more about sexual changes proceeding neurological and movement disorder in HD. Clearly, studies that incorporate both patients and their partner to obtain reliable information on their sexual life would be reasonable. Further investigation on the context of sexual dysfunction in association with neurophysiologic changes, depression, irritability and dementia symptoms are needed to better understand reasons for sexual changes in HD.

# 7. References

- AMERICAN PSYCHIATRIC ASSOCIATION, 1994. Diagnostic and Statistical Manual of Mental Disorders. *American Psychiatric Press. 4th ed. Washington D.C.*
- ARGIOLAS, A & MELIS, M.R, 2003. The neurophysiology of the sexual cycle. *J Endocrinol Invest*, 26, 20-22.
- AVASARALA, J.R, CROSS, A.H, TRINKAUS, K, 2003. Comparative assessment of Yale Single Question and Beck Depression Inventory Scale in screening for depression in multiple sclerosis. *Mult Scler,* 9, 307-310.
- BANCROFT, J, 1993. Impact of environment, stress, occupational, and other hazards on sexuality and sexual behavior. *Environ Health Perspect*, 101 Suppl 2, 101-107.
- BARTON, D, JOUBERT, L, 2000. Psychosocial aspects of sexual disorders. *Aust Fam Physician*, 29: 527-531.
- BEIER, K, GOECKER, D, BABINSKY, S, AHLERS, C, 2002. Sexualität und Partnerschaft bei Multipler Sklerose - Ergebnisse einer empirischen Studie bei Betroffenen und ihren Partnern. *Sexuologie*, 9, 4-22.
- BIRD, E.D, CHIAPPA, S.A, FINK, G, 1976. Brain immunoreactive gonadotropin-releasing hormone in Huntington's chorea and in non-choreic subjects. *Bird Nature*, 260, 536-538.
- BOERNER, R.J & KAPFHAMMER, H.P, 1999. Psychopathological changes and cognitive impairment in encephalomyelitis disseminata. *Eur Arch Psychiatry Clin Neurosci*, 249, 96-102.
- BOLT, J.M, 1970. Huntington's chorea in the West of Scotland. *Br J Psychiatry*, 116, 259-270.
- BONUCCELLI, U, NUTI, A; MAREMMANI, C, CERAVOLO, R, MURATORIO, A, 1992. Steroid therapy in Huntington's disease. *Adv Biochem Psychopharmacol*, 47, 149-154.
- BUCHANAN, R.J, WANG, S, TAI-SEALE, M, JU, H, 2003. Analyses of nursing home residents with multiple sclerosis and depression using the Minimum Data Set. *Mult Scler*, 9, 171-188.
- BURGENER, S, LOGAN, G, 1989. Sexuality concerns of the post-stroke patient. *Rehabil Nurs*, 14, 178-181
- BUVAT, J & LEMAIRE, A, 2001. Sexuality of the diabetic woman. *Diabetes Metab*, 27, 67-75.

- CALABRESE, P, 2006. Neuropsychology of multiple sclerosis, An overview. *J Neurol,* *253 Suppl* 1,i10-15.
- CHANDLER, B.J & BROWN, S, 1998. Sex and relationship dysfunction in neurological disability. *J Neurol Neurosurg Psychiatry*, 65, 877-880.
- CHANNON, L.D & BALLINGER, S.E, 1986. Some aspects of sexuality and vaginal symptoms during menopause and their relation to anxiety and depression. *Br J Med Psychol*, 59, 173-80
- CLAYTON, A.H, 2001. Recognition and assessment of sexual dysfunction associated with depression. *J Clin Psychiatry*, 62, 5-9.
- CRAUFURD, D, THOMPSON, J.C, SNOWDEN, J.S, 2001. Behavioral changes in Huntington Disease. *Neuropsychiatry Neuropsychol Behav Neurol*, 14, 219-226.
- CSESKO, P.A, 1988. Sexuality and multiple sclerosis. *J Neurosci Nurs,* 20, 353-355.
- DAKOF, G.A, TAYLOR, S.E, 1990. Victims' perceptions of social support: what is helpful from whom? *J Pers Soc Psychol*, 58, 80-89.
- DASGUPTA, R & FOWLER, C.J, 2003. Bladder, bowel and sexual dysfunction in multiple sclerosis: management strategies. *Drugs,* 63, 153-166.
- DE LOACH, D, GREER, B, 1981. Adjustment of severe physical disability: A metamorphosis. *McGraw Hill, New York.*
- DEWHURST, K, OLIVER J.E, MCKNIGHT A.L, 1970. Socio-psychiatric consequences of Huntington's disease. *Br J Psychiatry,* 116, 255-258.
- DRAGASITS, I, LEVINE, M.S, ZEITLIN, S, 2000. Inactivation of Hdh in the brain and testis results in progressive neurodegeneration and sterility in mice. *Nat Genet,* 26, 300-306.
- FAVA, M & RANKIN, M, 2002. Sexual functioning and SSRIs. *J Clin Psychiatry,* 63 Suppl 5, 13-16.
- FEDOROFF, J.P, PEYSER, C, FRANZ, M. L, FOLSTEIN, S.E, 1994. Sexual disorders in Huntington's disease. *J Neuropsychiatry Clin Neurosci*, 6, 147-153.
- FEINSTEIN, A & FEINSTEIN, K, 2001. Depression associated with multiple sclerosis, Looking beyond diagnosis to symptom expression. *J Affect Disord*, 66, 193–198.
- FEINSTEIN, A, FEINSTEIN, K, GRAY, T, O´CONNOR, P, 1997. Prevalence and neurobehavioral correlates of pathological laughing and crying in multiple sclerosis. *Arch Neurol,* 54, 1116-1121.

- FEINSTEIN, A, O'CONNOR, P, GRAY, T, FEINSTEIN, K, 1999. Pathological laughing and crying in multiple sclerosis: a preliminary report suggesting a role for the prefrontal cortex. *Mult Scler,* 5, 69-73.
- FOLEY, F & SANDERS, A, 1997. Sexuality, multiple sclerosis, and women. *MS Management,* 4, 1-10.
- FOWLER, C.J, 1997. The cause and management of bladder, sexual and bowel symptoms in multiple sclerosis. *Baillieres Clin Neurol,* 6, 447-466.
- FRUEHWALD, S, LOEFFLER, STASTKA, H, EHER, R, SALETU, B, BAUMHACKL, U, 2001. Depression and quality of life in multiple sclerosis. *Acta Neurol Scand,* 104, 257-261.
- GAGNE, P, 1981. Treatment of sex offenders with medroxyprogesterone acetate. *Am J Psychiatry,* 138, 644-646.
- GRAZIOTTIN, A, 1998. The biological basis of female sexuality. *Int Clin Psychopharmacol,* 13 Suppl 6, 15-22.
- GUNZELMANN, T, RUSCH, B.D, BRAHLER, E, 2004. Attitudes Towards Eroticism and Sexuality in the Elderly over 60 Years of Age. *Gesundheitswesen,* 66, 15-20.
- GÜTL, P, GREIMEL, E.R, ROTH, R, WINTER, R. 2002. Women's sexual behavior, body image and satisfaction with surgical outcomes after hysterectomy: a comparison of vaginal and abdominal surgery. *J Psychosom Obstet Gynaecol,* 23(1), 51-59.
- HAHLWEG, K, 1996. Fragebogen zur Partnerschaftsdiagnostik (FPD). Hogrefe-Verlag.
- HASSEBRAUCK, M, 1991. ZIP- Zufriedenheit in Paarbeziehungen- deutsche Fassung der Relationship Assessment Scale von Hendrick.
- HORDERN, A, 2000. Intimacy and sexuality for the woman with breast cancer. *Cancer Nurs,* 23, 230-236.
- HULTER, B.M, LUNDBERG, P,O 1995. Sexual function in women with advanced multiple sclerosis. *J Neurol Neurosurg Psychiatry,* 59, 83-86.
- HUNTINGTON, G, 1872. The Medical and Surgical Reporter. 26, 317-321.
- HUWS, R, SHUBSACHS, A.P, TAYLOE, P.J, 1991. Hypersexuality, fetishism and multiple sclerosis. *Br J Psychiatry,* 158, 280-281.
- JANARDHAN, V & BAKSHI, R, 2002. Quality of life in patients with multiple sclerosis: the impact of fatigue and depression. *J Neurol Sci,* 205, 51-58.
- JONSSON, A, 2003. Disseminated sclerosis and sexuality. *Ugeskr Laeger,* 165, 2642-2646.

- KALAYJIAN, L.A, MORRELL, M.J, 2000. Female sexuality and Neurological disease. *JSET*, 25, 89-95.
- KALB, R, 1998. Multiple sclerosis: A guide for families. *Demos Bermande, New York.*
- KAPLAN, S.A, REIS, R.B, KOHN, I.J, IKEGUCHI, E.F, LAOR, E, TE, A.E, MARTINS, A.C, 1999. Safety and efficacy of sildenafil in postmenopausal women with sexual dysfunction. *Urology,* 53, 481-486.
- KASPER, S, 2002. Sexuelle Dysfunktion bei depressiven Patienten. *Neurologie und Psychiatrie, Sonderausgabe April: 30.*
- KNEEBONE, II, DUNMORE, E.C, EVANS, E, 2003. Symptoms of depression in older adults with multiple sclerosis (MS): comparison with a matched sample of younger adults. *Aging Ment Health,* 7, 182-185.
- KOCH, T, KRALIK, D, EASTWOOD, S, 2002. Constructions of sexuality for women living with multiple sclerosis. *J Adv Nurs,* 39,137-145.
- KOCKOTT, G, 1989. Diagnostic and therapeutic possibilities in psychological disorders as a cause of impotence. Urologe, 28, 248-252.
- KOCKOTT, G & FAHRNER E-M, 2004. Sexualstörungen. *Thieme, Stuttgart.*
- KRUEGER, R.B & KAPLAN, M.S, 2001. Depot-leuprolide acetate for treatment of paraphilias: a report of twelve cases. *Arch Sex Behav,* 30, 409-422.
- LAAN, E, VAN LUNSEN, R.H, EVERAED, W, 2001. The effects of tibolone on vaginal blood flow, sexual desire and arousability in postmenopausal women. *Climacteric,* 4, 28-41.
- LANGE, H, 2002. Mb. Huntington, Diagnose und Therapie. *Psycho* 28, 479-486.
- LAUMANN, E.O, PAIK, A, ROSEN, R.C, 1999. Sexual dysfunction in the United States: prevalence and predictors. *Jama,* 281, 537-544.
- LEAVITT, B.R, GUTTMAN, J.A, HODGSON , J.G, KIMEL, G.H, SINGARAJA, R, VOGL, A.W, HAYDEN, M.R, 2001. Wild-type huntingtin reduces the cellular toxicity of mutant huntingtin in vivo. *Am J Hum Genet,* 68, 313-324.
- LEHMAN, D, HEMPHILL, K, 1990. Recipients' perceptions of support attempts and attributions for support attempts that fail. *Journal of Social and Personal Relationships,* 7, 563- 574.
- LILIUS, H.G, VALTONEN, E.J, WIKSTROM, J, 1976. Sexual problems in patients suffering from multiple sclerosis. *Scand J Soc Med,* 4, 41-44.
- LOEWIT, K, 2003. Position of sexual medicine in medical specialties. *Wien Med Wochenschr,* 153, 171-173.

- MARKIANOS, M, PANAS, M, KALFAKIS, N, VASSILOPOULUS, D, 2005. Plasma testosterone in male patients with Huntington's disease: relations to severity of illness and dementia. *Ann Neurol,* 57, 520-525.
- MATTSON, D, PETRIE, M, SRIVASTAVA, D.K, McDERMOTT, M, 1995. Multiple sclerosis. Sexual dysfunction and its response to medications. *Arch Neurol,* 52, 862-868.
- McCABE M, McDONALD E, DEEKS A, VOWELS L, COBAIN M, 1996. The impact of multiple sclerosis on sexuality and relationships. *Journal of Sex Research,* 33, 241.
- McCABE M.P, 2002. Relationship functioning and sexuality among people with multiple sclerosis. *J Sex Res,* 39, 302-309.
- McCABE, M.P, TALEPOROS, 2003. Sexual esteem, sexual satisfaction, and sexual behavior among people with physical disability. *Arch Sex Behav,* 32, 359-369.
- MCDONALD, W.I, COMPSTON, A, EDAN, G, GOODKIN, D, HARTUNG, H.P, LUBLIN, F.D, MCFARLAND, H.F, PARTY, D.W, ., CH, REINGOLD, S.C, SANDBERG-WOLLHEIM, M, SIBLEY, W, THOMPSON, A, VAN DEN NOORT, S, WEINSHENKER, B.Y, WOLINSKY, J.S, 2001. Recommended diagnostic criteria for multiple sclerosis: guidelines from the International Panel on the diagnosis of multiple sclerosis. *Ann Neurol, 50 (1),* 121-127.
- MCKEE, A.L. Jr, SCHOVER, L.R, 2001. Sexuality rehabilitation. *Cancer,* 92, 1008-1012.
- MINDEN, S.L & SCHIFFER, R.B, 1990. Affective disorders in multiple sclerosis. Review and recommendations for clinical research. *Arch Neurol,* 47, 98–104.
- MINDEN, S.L, 2000. Mood disorders in multiple sclerosis: diagnosis and treatment. *J Neurovirol, 6 Suppl 2,* 60-67.
- MINDEN, S.L, ORAV, J, REICH, P, 1987. Depression in multiple sclerosis. *Gen Hosp Psychiatry,* 9, 426-434.
- MONGA, T.N, TAN, G, OSTERMANN, H.J, MONGA, U, GRABOIS, M, 1998. Sexuality and sexual adjustment of patients with chronic pain. *Disabil Rehabil,* 20, 317-329.
- NEISES, M, 2002. Sexuality and Sexual Dysfunction in Gynecological Psychooncology. *Onkologie,* 25, 571-574.
- NELSON, L.D, ELDER, J.T, TEHRANI, P, GROOT, J, 2003. Measuring personality and emotional functioning in multiple sclerosis: a cautionary note. *Arch Clin Neuropsychol,* 18, 419-429.

- NICOLOSI, A, BUVAT, J, GLASSER, D.B, HARTMANN, U, LAUMANN, E.O, GINGELL, C, 2006. Sexual behaviour, sexual dysfunctions and related help seeking patterns in middle-aged and elderly Europeans: the global study of sexual attitudes and behaviors. *World J Urol,* 24, 423-428.
- NICOLOSI, A, MOREIRA, E.D. Jr, VILLA, M, GLASSER, D.B, 2004. A population study of the association between sexual function, sexual satisfaction and depressive symptoms in men. *J Affect Disord,* 82(2), 235-243.
- NUSBAUM, M.R, HAMILTON, C, LENAHAN, P, 2003. Chronic illness and sexual functioning. *Am Fam Physician,* 67, 347-354.
- OLIVER, J.E, 1970. Huntington's chorea in Northamptonshire. *Br J Psychiatry,* 116, 241-253.
- PANKSEPP, J, 2004. Textbook of Biological Psychiatry. *First edition, John Wiley and Sons,* New York, p 126.
- PAPALEXI, E, PERSSON, A, BJORKQVIST, M, PETERSEN, A, WOODMAN, B, BATES, GP, SUNDLER, F, MULDER, H, BRUNDIN, P, POPOVIC, N, 2005. Reduction of GnRH and infertility in the R6/2 mouse model of Huntington's disease. *Eur J Neurosci,* 22, 1541-1546.
- PATTEN, S.B, BECK, C.A, WILLIAMS, J.V, BARBUI, C, METZ, L.M, 2003. Major depression in multiple sclerosis: a population-based perspective. *Neurology,* 61, 1524-1527.
- PEREZ, M.A; SKINNER, E.C, MEYEROWITZ, B.E, 2002. Sexuality and intimacy following radical prostatectomy: patient and partner perspectives. *Health Psychol,* 21, 288-293.
- PIERINGER, W, 2007. "Psychodynamik und Psychosomatik". Psychotherapiewoche Bad Gleichenberg, PSY-III-Diplom. Vortrag.
- POLMAN, C.H, REINGOLD, S.C, EDAN, G, FILIPPI, M, HARTUNG, H.P, KAPPSOS, L, LUBLIN, F.D, METZ, L.M, MCFARLAND, H.F, O'CONNOR, P.W, SANDBERG-WOLLHEIM, M, THOMPSON, A.J, WEINSHENKER, B.G, WOLINSKY, J.S, 2005. Diagnostic criteria for multiple sclerosis: 2005 revisions to the "McDonald Criteria". *Ann Neurol,* 58 (6), 840-846.
- RICE, A, 2000. Sexuality in cancer and palliative care 1: Effects of disease and treatment. *Int J Palliat Nurs,* 6, 392-397.
- RICH, S.S & OVSIEW, F, 1994. Leuprolide acetate for exhibitionism in Huntington's disease. *Mov Disord,* 9, 353-357.

- ROSEN, R.C, RILEY, A, WAGNER, G, OSTERLOH, I.H, KIRKPATRICK, J, MISHRA, A, (1997) The international index of erectile function (IEEF): A multidimensional scale for assessment of erectile dysfunction. *Urology,* 49, 822–830.
- ROSEN, R, ALTWEIN, J, BOYLE, P, KIRBY, R.S, LUKACS, B, MEULEMAN, E, O'LEARY, M.P, PUPPO, P, ROBERTSON, C, GUILIANO, F, 2003. Lower urinary tract symptoms and male sexual dysfunction: the multinational survey of the aging male (MSAM-7). *Eur Urol,* 44, 637-649.
- SALEH, F.M & GUIDRY, L.L, 2003. Psychosocial and biological treatment considerations for the paraphilic and nonparaphilic sex offender. *J Am Acad Psychiatry Law,* 31, 486-493.
- SATHASIVAM, K, HOBBS, C, MANGIARINI, L, MAHAL, A, TURMAINE, M, DOHERTY, P, DAVIES, S.W, BATES, G.P, 1999. Transgenic models of Huntington's disease. *Philos Trans R Soc Lond B Biol Sci,* 354, 963-969.
- SCHMIDT, E.Z, HOFMANN, P, NIEDERWIESER, G, KAMPFHAMMER; H.P, BONELLI, R.M, 2005. Sexuality in multiple sclerosis. *J Neural Transm,* 112 (9), 1201-1211.
- SCHMIDT, E.Z, KAMPFHAMMER, H.P, BONELLI, R.M, 2007. Sexuality in Huntington's disease. *Wiener Med. Wochenzeitschrift*
- SCHMIDT, E.Z, REININGHAUS, B, HOFMAN, P 2006. Auffälligkeiten bei Patienten mit Multipler Sklerose. *Psychiatrie & Psychotherapie,* 2/1.
- SCHOVER, L.R, 1994. Sexuality and body image in younger women with breast cancer. *J Natl Cancer Inst Monogr,* 16, 177-182.
- SEIDMAN, S.N, 2002. Exploring the relationship between depression and erectile dysfunction in aging men. *J Clin Psychiatry, 63* Suppl 5, 5-12.
- SIMONS, J.S & CAREY, M.P, 2001. Prevalence of sexual dysfunctions: results from a decade of research. *Arch Sex Behav,* 30, 177-219.
- SJOGREN, K, DAMBER, J.E, LILIEQUIST, B, 1983. Sexuality after stroke with hemiplegia. I. Aspects of sexual function. *Scand J Rehabil Med,* 15, 55-61.
- SJOGREN, K, 1983. Sexuality after stroke with hemiplegia. II. With special regard to partnership adjustment and to fulfilment. *Scand J Rehabil Med,* 15, 63-69.
- SOLARI, A, MOTTA, A, MENDOZZI, L, ARIDON, P, BERGAMASCHI, R, GHEZZI, A, MANCARDI, G.L, MILANESE, C, MONTANARI, E, PUCCI, E, 2004. Italian version of the Chicago multiscale depression inventory: translation, adaptation and testing in people with multiple sclerosis. *Neurol Sci,* 24,375-383.

- STENAGER, E, STENAGER, E, JENSEN, K, BOLDSEN, J, 1990. Multiple sclerosis: Sexual dysfunctions. *Journal of Sex Education and Therapy,* 16, 262-269.
- STRAUß, B & RICHTER-APPELT, H 1996. The "Body Experience Questionnaire" "Fragebogen zur Beurteilung des eigenen Körpers"; FbeK. *Hogrefe, Göttingen*
- SZASZ G, PATY, D, LAWTON-SPEERT, S, EISEN K, 1984. A sexual functioning scale in multiple sclerosis. *Acta Neurologica Scandinavica* Supplement, 101, 37-43.
- TALLEY, C.L, 2005. The emergence of multiple sclerosis, 1870-1950: a puzzle of historical epidemiology. *Perspect Biol Med,* 48,383-395.
- VALLEROY, M.L, KRAFT, G.H, 1984. Sexual dysfunction in multiple sclerosis. *Arch Phys Med Rehabil,* 65, 125-128.
- VAN RAMMSDONK, J.M, PEARSON, J, ROGERS, D.A, BISSADA, N, VOGL, A.W, HAYDEN, M.R, LEAVITT, B.R, 2005. Loss of wild-type huntingtin influences motor dysfunction and survival in the YAC128 mouse model of Huntington disease. *Hum Mol Genet,* 14, 1379-1392.
- VAUGHIN, M.J & BAIER M.E.M 1999. Reliability and validity of the relationship assessment scale. *American Journal of Family Therapy,* 27 (2) April – June.
- VENTEGODT, S, 1996. Sexuality and quality of life. Results from the quality of life-study of 4,626 Danes aged 31-33 years born at Rigshospitalet 1959-1961. *Ugeskr Laeger,* 158, 4299-4304.
- VERMILLION, S, HOLMES, M, 1997. Sexual dysfunction in women. *Prom Care Update Ob/Gyns,* 4, 234-240.
- WEISSBACH-RIEGER, A, 1987. Partnership relations, sexuality and sexual behavior in elderly females and males after age 55. I. Partnership relations and sexuality from the social gynecologic and sociological viewpoint. *Zfa* 42, 203-205.
- ZEPHIR, H, DE SEZE, J, STOIJKOVIC, T, DELISSE, B, FERRIBY, D, CABARET, M, VERMERSCH, P, 2003. Multiple sclerosis and depression: influence of interferon beta therapy. *Mult Scler,* 9, 284-288.
- ZIMMER, D. 1989. Fragebogen zu Sexualität und Partnerschaft (ASP, TSST, NSP). 3. korr Auflage 1994, DGVT-Verlag.
- ZLOTTA, A.R & SCHULMANN, C.C, 1999. BPH and sexuality. *Eur Urol* 36 Suppl 1, 107-112.

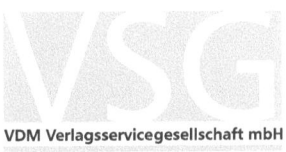

Die VDM Verlagsservicegesellschaft sucht für wissenschaftliche Verlage abgeschlossene und herausragende

## Dissertationen, Habilitationen, Diplomarbeiten, Master Theses, Magisterarbeiten usw.

für die kostenlose Publikation als Fachbuch.

Sie verfügen über eine Arbeit, die hohen inhaltlichen und formalen Ansprüchen genügt, und haben Interesse an einer honorarvergüteten Publikation?

Dann senden Sie bitte erste Informationen über sich und Ihre Arbeit per Email an *info@vdm-vsg.de*.

**Sie erhalten kurzfristig unser Feedback!**

VDM Verlagsservicegesellschaft mbH
Dudweiler Landstr. 99　　　　　Telefon  +49 681 3720 174
D - 66123 Saarbrücken　　　　　Fax　　　+49 681 3720 1749

**www.vdm-vsg.de**

Die VDM Verlagsservicegesellschaft mbH vertritt

 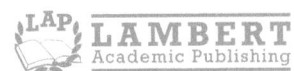 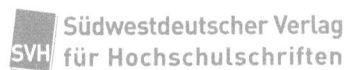

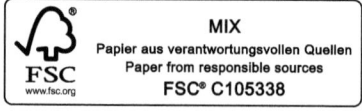

Printed by Books on Demand GmbH, Norderstedt / Germany